Regenerative Medicine

Building a Better, Healthier Body

By Theodore E. Harrison

MD MBA FACEP ABAARM

Acknowledgements

Many thanks to Charles Runels, MD, Sharon McQuillan, MD, and Kristin Comella, MS, our mentors and pioneers in the use of regenerative therapies in office practice. Their innovative ideas and research have pushed regenerative medicine out of the laboratory and into the community. I also owe a debt of gratitude to Durk Pearson and Sandy Shaw, who first introduced me to the idea of anti-aging medicine. And of course I want to thank my ever-patient wife, Louise Andrew, MD, who suffered through the preparation of this manuscript and helped edit parts of it.

Thanks are also due to my friends, family and colleagues who read through the draft versions and pointed out my errors and omissions. Particular thanks go to Drs. David Rabago, Lucretia van den Berg, Brian Shiple, Bryan Ward, Dan Morhaim, Jeff Weil, Federico Vasvari, Sonia Jones and Alexei Bagrov for their comments on the medical content. On the layperson side I have to thank Gail Corvette, Maria Hosmer, David Galland and Liz Worley for their comments on style and their help in editing and in identifying passages that needed revision in order to be intelligible to the general public.

Disclaimer

The information presented in this book is based on the experience and research of the author and is intended for informational and educational purposes only. Every effort has been made to ensure the accuracy and timeliness of the information presented; however, the field is advancing rapidly and we fully expect that some of the information contained in this book will be outdated even the day that the book is published. We encourage readers to do their own research to keep abreast of the current state of the art. Or you can follow our blog at www.rejuvacare.org.

It is not the purpose of this book to diagnose or treat medical problems. It is not a substitute for a physician's advice. Our legal obligation: The author shall have neither liability nor responsibility to any person or entity with respect to any loss or damage caused or alleged to be caused directly or indirectly by the information contained in this book. No medical decisions should be made based solely on the contents or recommendations made in this book.

If any information in this book appears to apply to your condition, we recommend that you get a formal evaluation by a physician who is competent in the area described.

Preface

Away from the spotlight of the evening news, a revolution in the treatment of many everyday medical problems is taking place. A lot of it doesn't even involve much high tech. No new drugs. Little in the way of innovative equipment. Hardly a computer in sight.

It's new knowledge that's driving the advance of regenerative medicine: knowledge about stem cells, growth factors, the human genome, hormones, and the wonderfully complex and interactive roles that all these things play in your body.

Our goal in this book is to educate consumers (and perhaps some physicians) in the ways that regenerative medicine is being used in medical practice today. I apologize in advance to the physicians for some of the elementary material included. Perhaps you can just skip it or use it to refresh your memory about platelets, stem cells, and embryology. I also apologize for the lack of citations in many instances. Much of this information derives from anecdotal personal experiences or data from press releases or conferences that just haven't made it into medical publications yet.

To the lay readers, I apologize for the use of specialized medical terminology. I have tried to detect and define all the terms used when they first occur so that you don't have to have a medical dictionary at hand while reading the book. I've also put them into a glossary at the end of the book for easy reference.

This book will be obsolete by the time you read it. The advances in regenerative medicine are coming so thick and fast that it's a challenge for a physician who practices it to keep up on a daily basis, let alone through such a static medium as a book. Just last year, 2014, we have witnessed dozens of new applications and hundreds of new studies advancing our knowledge in this new field of medicine.

However, there is a lot more to come. Despite the resistance of entrenched medical and governmental bureaucracies (who are always resistant to change), practitioners and researchers are pushing the boundaries every day. I suspect many of the techniques and procedures described in this book as cutting-edge today will be mainstream medical practice in just a few years. It's a great time to be alive and I hope that what you read here will make your life longer and better.

Contents

Part I:
What is
Regenerative
Medicine

1

Why Is It "Regenerative"?

Most people have never heard of regenerative medicine (also called cell medicine or cellular medicine), but they will. It's been more than two decades since Daniel Rudman published his seminal work on the effects of growth hormone on elderly men[1] —two decades that have witnessed an avalanche of research on hormones; the decoding of the human genome; and the gradual understanding of what stem cells can do and why they are so important. This flood of new information is now finally making its way into clinical practice and changing the lives of not just a handful of lucky research subjects, but millions of average people.

Regenerative medicine is the "process of replacing or regenerating human cells, tissues or organs to restore or establish normal function."[2] Basically it is the art of helping the body to heal itself using its own processes. Rather than drugs, which are usually used to kill, inhibit, or block organisms, cells, or processes, regenerative medicine uses natural hormones and body cells to restore normal anatomy, physiology and function. Instead of surgery, which usually removes parts of the body, regenerative medicine harnesses the growth factors and repair mechanisms intrinsic to the human body.

We're not prejudiced against drugs, chemotherapy, radiotherapy or surgery. All these mainstream medical treatments have their appropriate and useful places. Nor is regenerative medicine a magic cure-all that will suddenly replace all of medical knowledge that has built up over the centuries. Having said that, there are many medical problems for which conventional medicine still does not have an adequate solution. Some of those yet-unsolved problems can be better approached from a regenerative medicine perspective. They will be the subjects of this book.

Regenerative medicine, like emergency medicine, family medicine, and critical care medicine, is a specialty of breadth rather than depth. It applies to children as well as adults and the elderly. It applies to all organ systems and uses all diagnostic modalities. It applies to a wide variety of diseases. Its special area of knowledge is the application of the body's own natural processes to effect healing.

Let me give a few examples to illustrate. Chronic back pain can become very debilitating. Surgery is one approach to this problem. Medication is another. However the regenerative medicine approach is to use prolotherapy with platelet-rich plasma and perhaps stem cells. Bladder cancer may require surgery, but regenerative medicine can supply a replacement bladder from cells that will not be rejected by the recipient. Arthritis sufferers face eventual joint replacement or a lifetime of chronic pain. Regenerative medicine can make the surgery unnecessary while ameliorating the pain and restoring function.

2

How Does It Work?

It is, of course, complicated. Treating a problem using regenerative medicine techniques is not as simple as just prescribing an antibiotic or taking out a gall bladder. It's more like getting a complete tune-up of your car. You may change the oil, but you also need to adjust the spark plugs, tighten the fan belt, balance the tires, and top up the radiator fluid. All these things affect engine performance.

Of course, nothing in medicine is really a simple isolated problem. That infection for which you were prescribed an antibiotic could be trivial or life-threatening, depending on the state of your immune system, the presence of diabetes or cancer, or dozens of other factors. The difference is that regenerative medicine focuses on the other factors rather than on the antibiotic.

Two main therapeutic modalities used in regenerative medicine are stem cell and platelet-rich plasma (PRP, a cell therapy enhancer) therapy. Gene therapy will join these to form a triad in the near future. Ideally all three of these modalities are used simultaneously. In addition there are adjunctive modalities that help regeneration work, like biologics (hormones), delivery systems, and scaffolds.

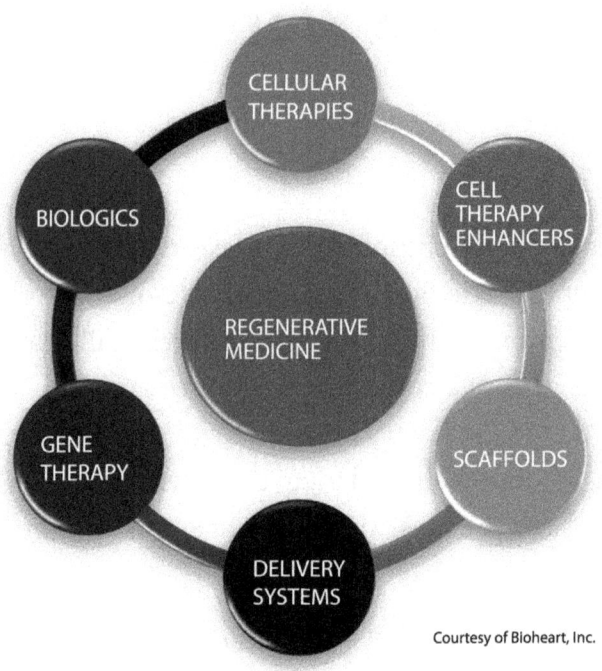

Courtesy of Bioheart, Inc.

Figure 1. Regenerative medicine comprises a number of areas.

Bioidentical Hormone Replacement Therapy (BHRT)

You could write a book (and many have been written already) on BHRT.[3,4,5,6] We are not going to reinvent the wheel here since others have done a far better job than we could do on the subject. Nonetheless we will try to give you an idea of why this is such an important aspect of regenerative medicine.

It's a sad fact of life that Mother Nature really only cares for us very much while we're growing up and producing children. Once the next generation is out of the womb, it's all about the grandkids and all downhill for the grandparents. In other words, your body does a great job of maintaining itself and staying healthy until your late twenties. After that, things gradually deteriorate.

There are a number of theories as to why this happens, but the important thing is to figure out what to do about it. One of the most obvious strategies is to replace things that wear out. Aubrey de Grey, a famous anti-aging researcher, has mapped out an entire strategy around this approach[7]. Regenerative medicine is an integral part of this strategy.

The first tactic adopted by many anti-aging physicians has been to try to keep hormone levels at their optimum—the levels we have in our late twenties. Since hormone levels are relatively easy to measure and natural replacement hormones are readily available, this is not

9

difficult to do. Unfortunately, hormone therapy has been given a bad reputation by people who have abused hormones and by drug companies whose artificial hormone products have backfired. However, there is considerable clinical evidence at this point that BHRT done right can mitigate the effects of aging.

This is important to regenerative medicine not only because it allows us to maintain body systems in better condition—keeping bones strong and preventing loss of muscle mass, for instance—but also because it provides an optimum therapeutic milieu for other interventions, such as stem cell therapies.

Let's face it. It's really hard to heal without adequate hormones. Thyroid hormone, testosterone, growth hormone, cortisone, and many other hormones play a vital role in homeostasis—keeping the body functioning properly. Estrogen, for instance, keeps women (and men) from having heart attacks. Vitamin D (yes, it's really a hormone) helps prevent osteoporosis. And the list goes on and on. You just can't be healthy without healthy hormone levels.

Of course this applies to your healing processes as well. That's why it's so important that anyone who is undergoing a stem cell or PRP treatment have normal, healthy hormone levels.

Platelet-Rich Plasma

What you see on the news is only the tip of the iceberg of what's going on in the field of stem cell therapy. The big stories are the dramatic ones about lives saved by organ replacement. Nevertheless, these dramatic procedures are still experimental and mostly a long way from becoming standard-of-care.

The behind-the-scenes story is what is going on today in doctors' offices around the world. That's what we're going to focus on in later chapters.

First; however, we're going to explain a little bit of the physiology—why these procedures work and how they can frequently reduce or eliminate the need for drugs or surgery. Here's the story:

When you are injured, say a little cut on your finger, the first thing that happens is that the platelets in your blood form a clot at the site of the cut to prevent you from losing blood.

What's a platelet? Platelets are "the smallest of the formed elements in blood, a disk-shaped, non-nucleated blood element with a fragile membrane, formed in the red bone marrow by fragmentation of megakaryocytes."[8] Platelets are like red blood cells, only smaller and without any hemoglobin in them. The megakaryocytes are big mother cells that live in the bone marrow. Little pieces of them break off; become platelets, and float off into the blood. Unlike cells, platelets don't have nuclei and can't replicate.

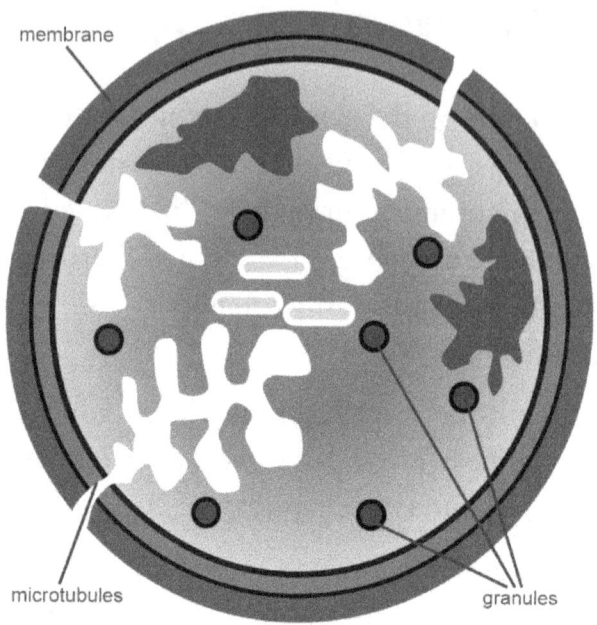

membrane

microtubules

granules

Figure 2. Platelets contain granules which release growth factors and cytokines.

Platelets (fig. 2) don't have much inner structure, but they do have organelles (little factories inside the platelet) and microtubules (long, thin little tubes inside the platelet which act kind of like a skeleton and muscles to maintain and change its shape). The organelles produce a big payload: three types of granules (each containing a unique batch of biologically active components) plus more than a thousand other chemicals such as cytokines (local signaling molecules—they carry information or instructions from one part of a cell to another or between cells) and growth factors (molecules which act on other cells to induce them to grow in specific ways). The most common growth factors include:

VEGF—Vascular Endothelial Growth Factor: helps build new blood vessels

bFGF—Basic Fibroblast Growth Factor: helps build new tissue cells, especially connective tissue

EGF—Epidermal Growth Factor: helps build new skin

TGF—Transforming Growth Factor: helps tissue development and regeneration

PDEGF—Platelet-derived Epidermal Growth Factor: another tissue builder

IGF—Insulin-like Growth Factor: A growth-regulating molecule induced by growth hormone

PDGF—Platelet-derived Growth Factor: regulates blood vessel formation

Normally platelets just float around in blood doing nothing. But when they encounter damage in a blood vessel wall, they swing into action. First they become activated. They lose their smooth discoid shape and become spiky and sticky (fig. 3). They stick to everything around them (like red blood cells, white blood cells, other platelets) and this is what forms the blood clot. This is just the first stage.

PLATELETS

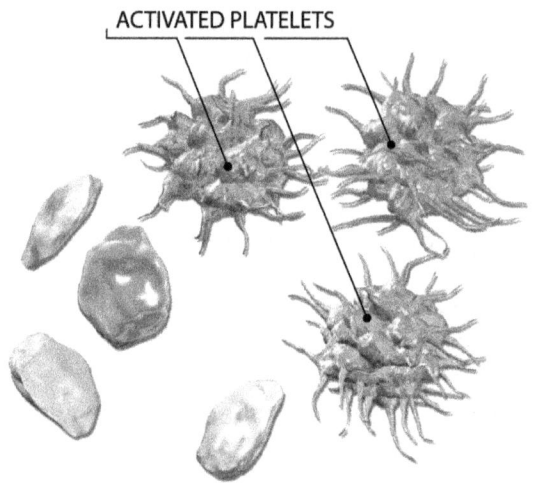

Figure 3. Activated platelets get spiky and sticky.

The blood clot will dissolve in a day or two, so the platelets have to do something to turn the temporary bandage into a permanent repair. They dump their granules and secrete growth factors and cytokines into the surrounding tissue. These molecules do many jobs. They help clean up dead cells and debris; help prevent infection; attract stem cells, which divide and supply new cells to replace damaged ones; and cause new blood vessels to grow to supply oxygen and nutrients to the freshly grown tissue. In addition, the platelets stick to receptors on other cells and send signals to their nuclei, which causes their DNA to produce new proteins that assist in the healing process.

After the initial burst of activity the platelets continue to make and secrete their growth and reconstruction factors for the rest of their brief lifespan—5 to 9 days. The stem cells take over at this point and continue the healing process. Eventually the damage is repaired and the tissue is almost as good as new (fig. 4).[9]

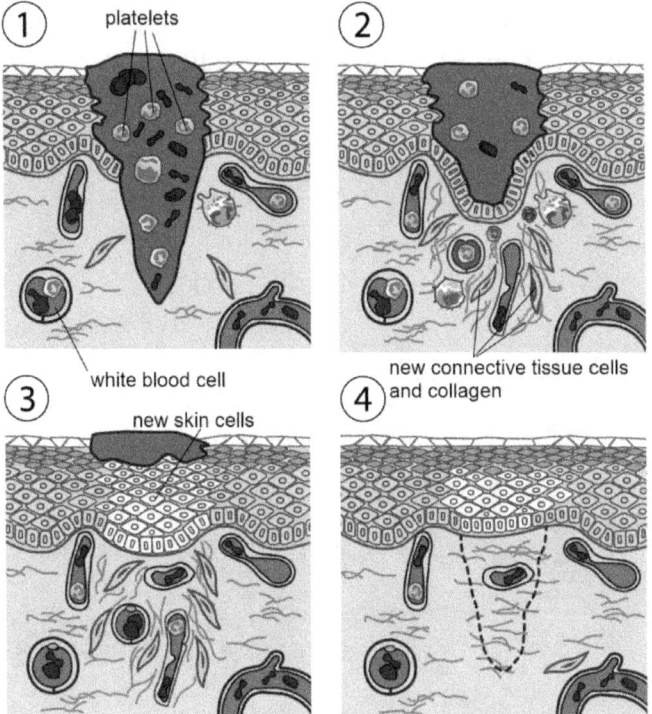

Figure 4. 1. Platelets form a clot. 2. Stem cells grow into it to repair tissue. 3. The dermis regrows (under a scab). 4. The epidermis heals and scab falls away.

We can harness this platelet regenerative activity to help heal parts of the body other than blood vessels. It turns out that the growth factors and cytokines in platelets have the same effect virtually everywhere. So we can take platelets from the blood, inject them where they are needed, and induce the same sort of reaction that occurs when a blood vessel is cut.

The first step in this process is to isolate and concentrate the platelets. We do this by drawing some blood; centrifuging it so that it separates out into layers; and then drawing off the layer where the platelets are concentrated (fig. 5). This layer is called the platelet-rich plasma, or PRP.

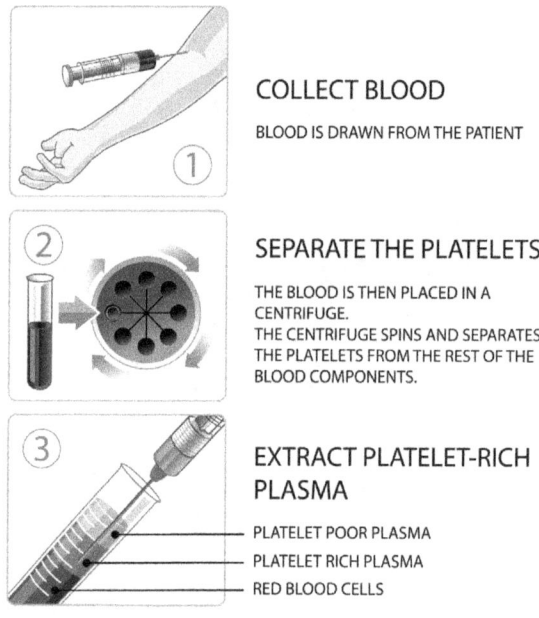

COLLECT BLOOD

BLOOD IS DRAWN FROM THE PATIENT

SEPARATE THE PLATELETS

THE BLOOD IS THEN PLACED IN A CENTRIFUGE.
THE CENTRIFUGE SPINS AND SEPARATES THE PLATELETS FROM THE REST OF THE BLOOD COMPONENTS.

EXTRACT PLATELET-RICH PLASMA

PLATELET POOR PLASMA
PLATELET RICH PLASMA
RED BLOOD CELLS

Figure 5. PRP is prepare by centrifuging a tube of blood and drawing off the platelet-rich layer.

We can activate the platelets by adding a little calcium to the PRP and this turns on the release of those important growth factors and cytokines. Then we can inject the activated PRP into damaged or diseased tissue and let the platelets go about their regenerative work: recruiting stem cells to the area and inducing new tissue growth.

PRP has been around since the 1950s, but its healing properties were not really recognized until the mid 1980s when first surgeons, then dentists, and then other medical specialties began to publish reports of its effectiveness. Now virtually every specialty has found a use for it and it is used to enhance everything from cardiac surgery recovery to the healing of skin ulcers.

Stem Cells

What's a stem cell? It's a cell that specializes in producing new cells. There are many different types, ranging from embryonic stem cells (the very first ones, from which your whole body is eventually formed) to adult stem cells (in an adult, stem cells become more specialized and every tissue type has its own different stem cells). It may surprise you to learn that all the new cells in your body come from your adult stem cells, and these are only a small fraction of all cells. Most mature adult cells are unable to divide and make new cells. So every organ and tissue has its own special stem cells that rush to the scene of an emergency just like an ambulance to an accident.

However, this does not mean that a fat stem cell, for instance, can produce only more fat cells. Stem cells are quite flexible and we now know that some adult stem cells can produce a diverse array of tissues.

Pericytes (top center in fig. 6)) are stem cells that occur throughout the body wrapped around blood vessels and capillaries. They monitor the blood for signals of injury. When they detect injury-related chemicals in the blood they turn into mesenchymal stem cells (MSCs) and enter the blood stream to home in on the injury. Once there, they can differentiate into any of a wide variety of tissue types depending on what is needed.

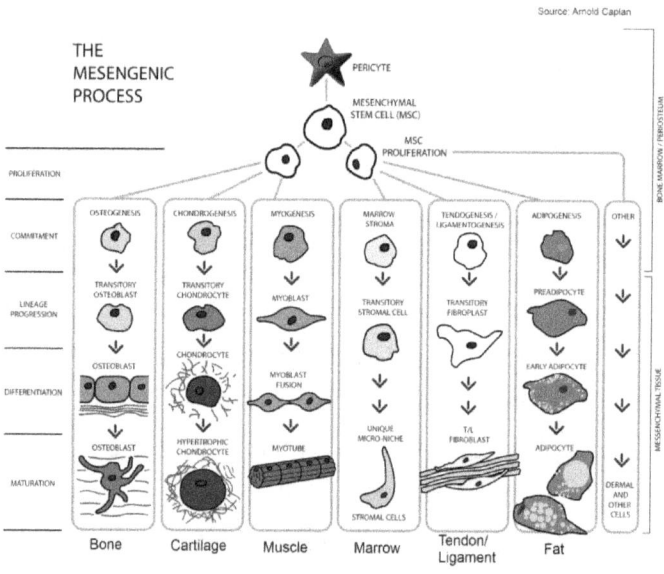

Figure 6. Stem cells "grow up" to become all the different tissues and organs of the body.

Not only that, but scientists have now developed techniques to reverse differentiation, so that we can make stem cells from already-mature cells. These are called induced Pluripotent Stem Cells (iPSCs). It's not clear yet whether these stem cells will be as good as natural stem cells in healing and repair.

The main purpose of stem cells is to duplicate themselves and provide new cells of the types needed to repair damage. When damage to a tissue occurs, stem cells rush to the scene to provide the bricks and mortar for repairs. However, they also secrete many of the same growth factors as platelets (and probably others as well). It is the growth factors and other proteins that act as the managers of the repair project. They direct the stem cells, determining where they will go and how they will create which kinds of cells so that well-organized functional tissue is produced.

One of the main differences between platelets and stem cells, however, is that stem cells stick around and reproduce themselves. Platelets are short-lived and are quickly used up. They deliver their payloads for a few days and they're done. Stem cells do their job and keep on going. They not only secrete the growth factors necessary for tissue repair, but also create new tissue cells, more extracellular matrix (the stuff that holds everything together), and copies of themselves for future use. Because they are fully functional cells, they express new proteins and communicate with each other.

It's the managerial capabilities of the stem cells and platelets that regenerative medicine harnesses in the procedures described in later chapters. Placing stem cells into areas where damage repair is needed can result in an influx of more cells, reorganization of the tissue, and restoration of function.

This is a two-stage process. The first stage is called *immunomodulatory*. It's when the cells signal to each other and recruit new cells. We see the symptoms of this as inflammation. It usually lasts a week or two.

The second stage is called *trophic*. During this time the cells divide and organize themselves into new tissue. It's mostly finished in about six weeks, but continues at a lower level for six months to a year or even longer. The process is so gradual that you can't see anything happening on a day-to-day basis, but photos and functional test measurements taken before and after will show significant improvements.

Why do we need to add or stimulate stem cells? Why doesn't the body just handle it on its own? When we are young it does. But as we age our stem cells also age. They don't work quite so well and they don't home in on areas of trouble as efficiently (fig. 7). We can help the body perform its regeneration by giving it new stem cells where they are needed.

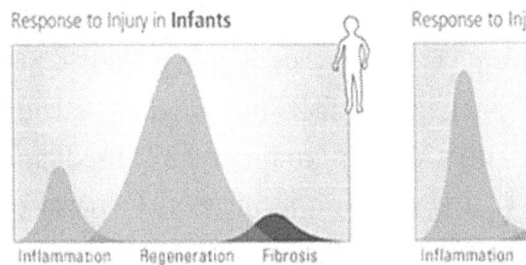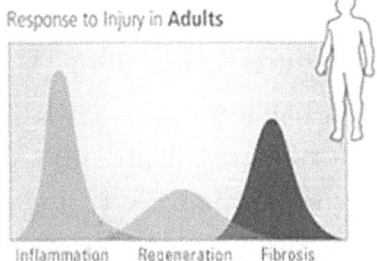

Figure 7. Infants have lots of highly functional stem cells and heal rapidly with little inflammation. Adults have fewer stem cells and don't respond as well (charts by Osiris Therapeutics, Inc.).

Prolotherapy

Prolotherapy (short for "proliferative therapy") is a technique developed by an American surgeon, Dr. George Hackett, in the 1940s and 1950s. In short, it is a method for strengthening and repairing ligaments, tendons, joint capsules, and their attachments to bones. It involves the injection of a small amount of a proliferative solution, usually 15–25% dextrose (a type of sugar), into the affected area. Dr. Hackett did a number of animal and human studies which showed that this technique worked to alleviate many painful skeletal conditions: back pain, whiplash injury, and tennis elbow, among others. His[10] and other animal research has shown that prolotherapy "significantly increases bone-ligament-bone junction strength and ligament mass and thickness when compared to saline-injected controls."[11]

Prolotherapy was popular for a while, but its fortunes faded when early adopters had some complications and more complex (and highly reimbursable) orthopedic procedures came along. However, in recent years it has been making a comeback.[12,13] In fact, it has gotten strong endorsement from no less a mainstream medicine personage than Dr. C. Everett Koop, Surgeon General of the United States during the Reagan years, who wrote, *"When I was 40 years old, I was diagnosed in two separate neurological clinics as having intractable (incurable) pain. My comment was that I was too young to have intractable pain. It was by chance that I learned that Gustav A. Hemwall, M.D., a practitioner in the suburbs of Chicago, was an expert in Prolotherapy. When I asked him if he could cure my pain, he asked me to describe it. When I had done the best that I could, he replied, 'There is no such pain. Do you mean a pain...' And then he continued to describe my pain much better than I could. When I said, "That's it exactly," he said, "I can fix you." To make a long story short, my intractable pain was not intractable and I was remarkably improved to the point where my pain ceased to be a problem. Much milder recurrences of that pain over the next 20 years were re-treated the same way with equally beneficial results."*

The fact that prolotherapy undoubtedly works has kept a strong cadre of active practitioners around. It even has its own foundation (The Hackett-Hemwall Foundation, http://www.hackethemwall.org) and is an integral part of the Family Medicine Residency program at the University of Wisconsin, which puts on a training program each year. Several good books have been written on prolotherapy lately, including *Prolo Your Pain Away*,[14] and *Prolotherapy: The Hollywood Pain Solution*[15] In fact, Dr. Hackett's original book, now in its third edition, is still in print: *Ligament and Tendon Relaxation (Skeletal Disability) Treated by Prolotherapy (Fibro-osseous Proliferation).*[16]

Lately, with the arrival of PRP and stem cell therapies, there has been a surge of interest in new techniques of prolotherapy.[17] It appears that the combination of prolotherapy methods with PRP and/or stem cell proliferative solutions may result in even better outcomes than traditional prolotherapy. Instead of relying on a passive proliferative solution like dextrose to cause mild inflammation and attract stem cells to the treatment area, this new model uses a solution like PRP that contains active growth factors that start the regenerative process, or stem cells themselves, which immediately start rebuilding. With this extra boost, prolotherapy can accomplish things that required major surgery in the past and treatment times are cut significantly. In later chapters we'll cover some of these procedures in detail.

Lasers and Radiofrequency

Since they destroy tissue, you might not think of lasers or radio frequency as regenerative modalities. But they do share the same basic mechanism as other regenerative methods—stimulating your own stem cells to produce new tissue. Here's how it works:

Lasers and radiofrequency waves are both the same thing - electromagnetic radiation (EMR). The difference between them is in the frequency of the EMR. Visible light spans the frequency range from ultraviolet to infrared, and includes many different frequencies mixed together. Lasers narrow the light down to a single frequency. You might call this a "pure" color. Radios use the same EMR but at lower frequencies than light. Microwave ovens use EMR that is between radio and infrared on the frequency spectrum.

EMR is transformed into heat energy when it is absorbed by certain substances. This, of course, is how microwave ovens work. But radio and light frequency EMR can also be used this way. Different frequencies penetrate the skin to different depths and are absorbed and transformed into heat by different substances. Water, hemoglobin, hair, and skin pigment, for instance, all absorb different frequencies.

So the technique of EMR treatment is the science of matching up a target substance at a particular depth at or below the skin surface with an appropriate frequency and dose. When this is done precisely, heat is generated in the target tissue. This causes changes in the tissue which may range from molecular rearrangement to complete cell destruction. The process in all cases, however, causes some degree of inflammation. Inflammation causes local stem cells to release their growth factors and start replication. Simultaneously the stem cells send signals to attract other stem cells to the area to help out. The final result is the remodeling and growth of new tissue in the area.

Let's look at a couple of examples. Laser therapy can be used to remove tattoos. Tattoos consist of colored pigments which have been taken up by skin cells. Because the pigment is inside the cells, the only way to get rid of a tattoo is to get rid of the cells that contain the pigment. If a laser of the right frequency is directed at tattooed cells of a particular color, the energy will cause those cells to heat up and die. The dead cells, along with the tattoo pigment, will then be reabsorbed by the body. Most cell parts will be recycled, but tattoo pigment, having no useful purpose, will be excreted. New skin cells from the endogenous (already there in the skin) skin stem cells will replace the old ones. The tattoo will disappear. (Because tattoos frequently are in several colors, several wavelengths and often several treatments may be required).

Radiofrequency (RF) EMR can be used to tighten up loose skin. One of the problems we face as we age is that our skin becomes "looser." Some of this is due to loss of subcutaneous tissue support, but some is due to the structure of the skin itself. Much of skin and the subcutaneous tissue consists of a molecule called collagen. Collagen is a fibrous protein material that stretches throughout the skin and subcutaneous tissue like a loosely woven blanket surrounding the fat cells, skin cells, capillaries, and other skin components and holding them all together and supporting the smooth surface we were born with. With age, collagen tends to gradually degrade and lose its strength and elasticity, allowing sagging to occur and wrinkles to form.

The application of heat can cause the collagen fibers to rearrange their structure and to contract. This causes the skin to tighten up with anywhere from 30 to 70% surface area reduction. If temperature at the surface is properly controlled, RF does not cause any visible scarring, but probably does stimulate fibroblast (connective tissue) stem cells, which make new cells and new collagen for the area. In radio frequency EMR treatments a RF probe is applied to the surface of the skin or inserted under the skin (or both) and RF EMR is applied. RF at a specific frequency for a specific time can produce temperatures of 40–50 degrees (Centigrade) in the subcutaneous tissue. This is enough to cause collagen reorganization in the (dermis and subcutaneous) tissue without damaging the overlying skin. The result is some immediate tightening of the skin with subsequent reorganization and concomitant reduction or disappearance of fine wrinkles. This appearance will mature over the next few months as the inflammation and proliferation runs its course, but the effects are essentially permanent (subject to continuing ordinary aging) as far as we know at this time.

In the same way, laser frequency EMR can be applied to the surface of the skin. If the frequency/dose is in an "ablative" (highly damaging) range, the skin cells will be destroyed. Growth factors are then released; stem cells are recruited; and the skin will regrow over a period of a couple of weeks. Newer laser modalities can ablate skin in defined patterns, leaving intact skin between the islands of ablation. Using this type of laser (called "fractional"), the adjacent skin cells contribute to filling the islands with stem cells and growth factors. The skin heals much more quickly, typically in 3 to 5 days.

Of course these aren't the only uses for lasers or radio frequency. But you get the idea: targeted heat can cause remodeling and regrowth of tissues.

Part II: Regenerative Procedures in the Medical Office

3

Aesthetic Procedures

It seems that people are more willing to pay for beauty than for their health. So it's not surprising that many of the first regenerative medical procedures were cosmetic. In this chapter we'll explain a number of state-of-the-art regenerative medical procedures that may replace traditional surgical or medical aesthetic procedures.

Facelift and Facial

"Tim and I stopped in the airport restaurant while waiting for our flight. When I ordered a glass of wine they carded me! LOL"

Ginger M., 55-year-old teacher,
one day after her "Vampire Facelift™."

Aging is seen earliest in the face. As we grow older we gradually lose some of the fat, subcutaneous tissue, and even bone in our facial structure. We *don't* lose any of the overlying skin, so it becomes loose, saggy, and wrinkled. The traditional approach to this problem is to tighten up the skin by removing small strategic areas and pulling the skin taut over the face. This method involves major surgery with its attendant risks and downtime, not to mention the expense. The results are frequently quite good in skilled hands, but the resulting appearance may not be quite natural.

There are several regenerative medicine approaches to the loss of facial skin tension, and they all center on restoring the volume of the face rather than removing skin. The least invasive of these (used on people with the least volume loss) is laser regenerative therapy. Laser light can reach deep enough into the skin to stimulate fibroblasts to produce more collagen. At the same time they can cause existing collagen to tighten up. So there is a combination of more volume with less skin, leading to the smoothing of wrinkles.

The simplest invasive procedure is the PRP facial[18] (sometimes called the vampire facial,[19,20] but not the same as the Vampire Facelift™). In this procedure, PRP is applied directly to the facial skin, sometimes with the aid of a needle roller or dermapen to make small holes in the skin through which the PRP can be better absorbed. The PRP reaches the subcutaneous tissue layer and there stimulates cell growth of both subcutaneous tissue and skin cells. This results in a remodeling of the skin with new blood vessels, thicker, more glowing skin with better color, and reduction in fine wrinkles.

A more advanced technique is called the "Vampire Facelift.™(www.vampirefacelift.com) "[21] In this technique doctors use both PRP and hyaluronic acid (HA) filler. HA is a normal, natural component of subcutaneous tissue. It is found all over the body, especially in skin, connective tissue, and joints, where it provides lubrication and shock absorption. HA loves water and absorbs and binds large amounts relative to its volume. It helps keep our tissues well lubricated and hydrated. However, like collagen, it's one of the things that we lose as we age.

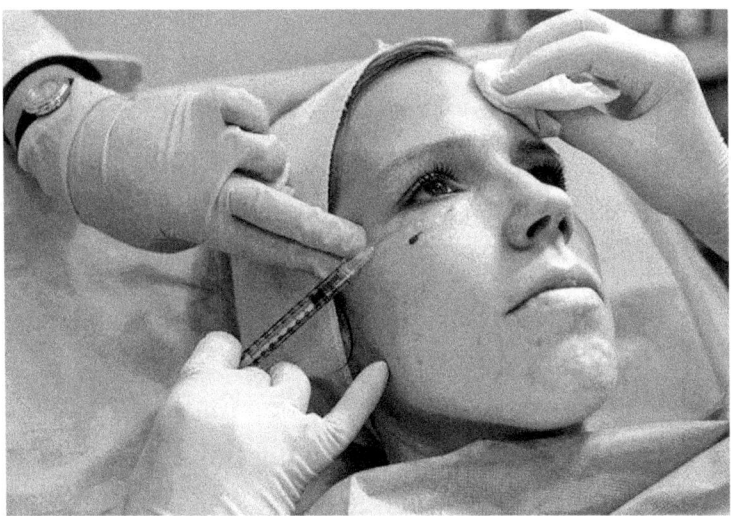

Figure 8. The vampire facelift involves the injection of PRP and HA under the skin of the face.

In the Vampire Facelift™ doctors inject HA and then PRP in strategic locations around the face to bring back the volume that has been lost with age (fig. 8). This pushes up the overlying skin, smoothing out wrinkles and folds. On its own the HA would gradually be absorbed by the body and the effects would be temporary. However, the HA attracts water and acts as a scaffolding for the subcutaneous and fat stem cells, which are attracted by the PRP. The stem cells divide and create new subcutaneous tissue resulting in improved facial volume and a younger look. As an added bonus, the PRP also acts as it does in the PRP facial, improving facial skin tone, strength, texture, and color.

Autologous fat grafting is another way of doing the same thing. In this method, rather than relying on PRP to attract stem cells, physicians do a small liposuction procedure and harvest stem cells directly from the patient's own fat. Then they inject both the fat and the stem cells into the appropriate locations on the face to increase the subcutaneous volume. Some practitioners add PRP during this procedure too.

The result is similar to the Vampire Facelift™—the facial skin is uplifted and wrinkles and folds are smoothed. The enhancing effect on the overlying skin is also similar.

The choice between the two— whether the Vampire Facelift™ or autologous fat graft is right for a particular patient—is both an economic and an aesthetic one. The Vampire Facelift™ is quicker, less complicated, and less expensive. However it achieves its best results in patients with only mild facial volume loss and becomes much more expensive when large volumes are required: the costs of HA and PRP are volume-dependent. Autologous fat grafts work best with patients who need moderate to large replacement of facial fat (generally older patients). The cost for a fat graft is usually fairly constant, so it doesn't make much difference how much volume is required.

Snoreplasty

It's said that about one-fifth of the adult population snores and that the fraction increases to 60% in men over the age of 40. It's a frequent topic of marital discord and may be a sign of obstructive sleep apnea. There are many devices, procedures, surgical operations and other remedies for snoring, but there is no consensus on what is best. In actuality, there is probably not a one-size-fits-all "best" solution as every patient is different and there are a number of different causes of snoring.

However, the most frequent cause (estimated at more than eighty percent) of snoring is palatal flutter—the soft palate in the roof of the mouth becomes lax and air movement through the mouth and nose during sleep causes it to vibrate, making the characteristic sounds. Injection snoreplasty is a simple treatment introduced in 2001[22] in which patients with palatal fluttering are given an injection of a sclerosant (a chemical that causes scarring) under topical anesthesia into the soft palate. This takes only a few minutes. The sclerosant causes scarring, and hence stiffening, of the soft palate in about 6 to 8 weeks. The stiff soft palate does not vibrate as much and snoring is greatly reduced in most cases.

A more recent, regenerative, version of this procedure has been developed,[23] in which PRP and/or other growth-stimulating solutions are used instead of a sclerosing agent. The outcome is the same (decreased snoring), but the PRP stimulates stem cells and induces the growth of normal connective tissue rather than scar tissue. The procedure is therefore more physiologically "natural." It also avoids even the very few and very minor complications of sclerosant therapy.

Since the injection snoreplasty procedure is so simple and inexpensive, and has minimal side effects or risks, some have advocated using it as a diagnostic test[24] rather than having the patient go through sleep studies, nasopharyngeal endoscopy, or other procedures to determine whether snoring is of palatal fluttering origin or not. If the patient responds well to the procedure then the diagnosis and treatment are both accomplished in one step. If they do not, then other causes can be sought.

The use of injection snoreplasty to treat sleep apnea is still in the early stages of investigation. A couple of pilot studies have been done, but since sleep apnea is a much more complicated problem than simple snoring it seems unlikely that snoreplasty by itself will prove to be a cure. Nor does the fact that snoring has been cured by snoreplasty mean that sleep apnea has been cured. If there are still signs and symptoms of sleep apnea a complete workup is indicated.

Breast Lift and Augmentation

Breast augmentation as a surgical procedure has been around for decades. Breast augmentation using autologous fat transfer has been tried for about 15 years. So there is little that's really new about this procedure except the use of regenerative medicine technique.

In classical breast augmentation, an incision is made in the breast and an implant, similar to a small balloon filled with jelly, is inserted underneath the breast tissue and sewn onto the chest wall. This is a major surgical procedure and requires general anesthesia and post-op time in the hospital. Like all major surgery, it has potential complications.

You would think that taking fat from where it's not wanted and putting it where it is wanted would be an easy procedure. However it took quite a while to figure out how to do this successfully. Surgeons have been experimenting with this for decades, but there were always two big problems: 1) Fat doesn't graft easily. Fat is very vascular (has many blood vessels), but unlike many major organs like kidneys and hearts, the blood vessels are very small. There is no way to reconnect the arteries and veins of a piece of fat in a new place in the body. Thus the transplanted fat cells usually just die off. 2) Obtaining fat is not all that simple, either. Removing fat surgically gives you large pieces of tissue that won't take in a graft (see #1, above). Liposuction has been used more successfully, but it developed a reputation for bleeding complications (because of all those small blood vessels).

The successful solution is a technique called tumescent liposuction. In this method, a local anesthetic solution is infused into an area of excess fat. This makes the area numb and also inhibits bleeding and facilitates liposuction. The solution is sucked back out along with fat cells through a small cannula. The fat cells are then separated from each other and from the anesthetic fluid. Stem cells can be separated from a portion of the fat cells by centrifugation, and then added back to the remaining fat cells to produce a stem-cell-rich fat graft.

The stem-cell-rich, autologous (donor and recipient are the same person) fat is not just inserted into the breast in one lump like an implant. Even with the extra stem cells, there wouldn't be enough blood supply for the graft to survive. Instead, the fat is injected back into the breast in thin tracks and in several layers. This way the new cells are always near a blood vessel. The stem cells secrete growth factors that promote the growth of new capillaries into the transplanted fat so that within a few days the transplanted fat cells are receiving adequate nourishment from the blood. Therefore, while some transplanted cells will still die, most will survive, and the breast will retain most of the volume added after the transplant (fig. 9).

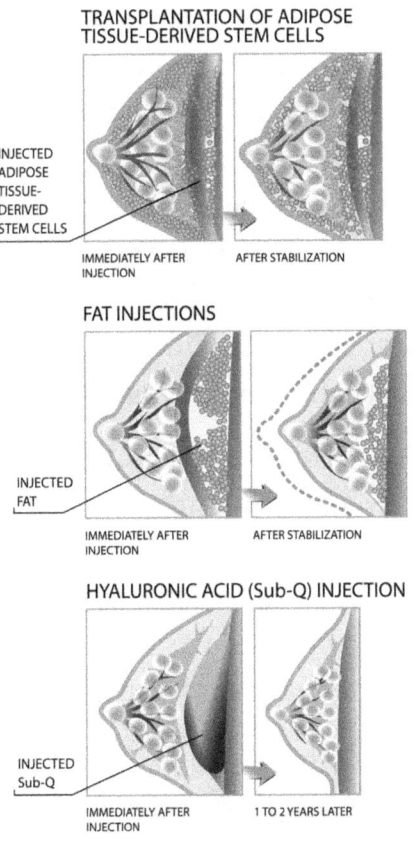

Figure 9. Breast augmentation with a stem cell fat graft (top pair of drawings) gives a much better result than with fat graft alone (middle) or filler (bottom).

The actress Suzanne Somers had this procedure done to restore one of her breasts after a battle with breast cancer. She wrote a book about the experience[25] and is now an active advocate of stem cell therapy.

The Breast Lift is a relatively minor non-surgical procedure (www.vampirebreastlift.com) that adds only a little volume to the breast, but is used to enhance the contour of the cleavage so as to present a more attractive décolletage. It uses a combination of HA and PRP to round out the upper inner aspect of a breast. This gives somewhat the same effect as a pushup bra and is frequently used after implants or age has caused some atrophy and flattening in this area. As in other places where HA and PRP are used together, the result is that new tissue is formed over time on the HA scaffolding resulting in rejuvenation of the original convex contours.

As an added bonus during this procedure, PRP is frequently injected into the areola, which can push the nipple out and cure inverted nipples; and PRP is also injected beneath the areola, which can result in the return of nipple sexual sensation, the loss of which is not an unusual complication of implant surgery.

Buttock Augmentation

Sometimes called the Brazilian Butt Lift, augmentation of the buttocks is very popular in Latin America and becoming more so in North America. The problems involved and the techniques to solve them are very similar to those of breast augmentation. As you might expect, however, even more volume may be required. This can be challenging in thin people, as they may simply not have enough fat.

There are a couple of potential solutions to this problem: 1) harvest fat from other areas in addition to the abdomen—flanks, thighs, and back frequently have fat reservoirs that can be tapped; 2) have the patient go on a short-term high-fat diet. Once they've put on about ten pounds the excess fat will make it much easier to harvest an adequate amount. This is one of the few times you'll ever see a doctor recommend ice cream as an important part of your diet!

Hands

Like the face, the hands suffer from a gradual loss of fatty subcutaneous tissue as they age. The back of the hands begin to show veins more prominently and fine wrinkles appear. The skin becomes thin and weak and perhaps discolored.

Also like the face, the hands respond well to autologous fat grafting. It's fairly easy to replace the thin layer of fat under the skin. The fat is harvested by liposuction and then enhanced with stem cells and PRP. It is then injected under the skin of the back of the hand and squeezed around under the skin until evenly distributed. As you might expect the increase in volume supports the overlying skin and smooths out wrinkles while obscuring veins.

The growth factors also have the expected effects on the skin, which improves in tone, color, strength, and thickness. There may even be a little spillover pain-relief effect on hand arthritis, if present.

For people with just fine wrinkles on the backs of the hands laser regeneration may add enough volume to do the job while also tightening the skin.

Neck

The skin under the chin at the front of the neck also loses support over time and becomes loose and flabby. In men, particularly, it may become reddened and rough, the so-called "rooster neck." At the same time, excess fat may occur in parts of the neck causing double chin or loss of definition of the chin.

This is a particularly difficult area, and may need minor liposuction in some places, fat transplant in other places and PRP or radiofrequency treatment in yet others. The objective is to tighten up the skin while, at the same time, removing wrinkles and improving the color, tone, and texture of the skin.

Scars

Case Report

A 55-year old woman presented with a large (~6cm²) depression in the skin of her forehead surrounded by discolored irregular scar tissue. This was secondary to the removal of a skin cancer from the area. She had been told by her plastic surgeon that nothing more could be done.

The scar tissue was treated with intradermal PRP and later on, at a second visit, the depressed area was treated with a slurry of PRP and hyaluronic acid. After a few weeks the scar tissue smoothed out and became more naturally colored and the depressed area more closely approached the level of the surrounding skin.

Scarring is how the body usually heals trauma. It can also happen after surgery, acne, piercings, or even cortisone therapy. The purpose is to quickly regain the integrity of the skin in order to prevent infection and the loss of bodily fluids. However, in its haste to get the defect patched, the body sometimes does a poor job of healing. Scar tissue is composed of the same material (collagen) as normal subcutaneous tissue, but it is denser and more uniformly aligned. This leaves the scarred area weaker and causes inhibition of normal regeneration of the skin, including loss of sweat glands and hair. Sometimes there is discoloration of the scar. Frequently collagen is overexpressed in the scar, which leads to either a raised or depressed area of scar tissue.

Sometimes laser therapy will help scars, especially smaller and/or pigmented ones. As in face and hand skin rejuvenation, the laser light can penetrate deep enough to stimulate the fibroblasts to produce new collagen and to reorganize the tissue of the scar.

It is not unusual to find that PRP therapy can help remodel scars where treatments like surgery, lasers, dermabrasion or skin peels have failed. As in other tissues, PRP releases growth factors into the dense scar tissue. This seems to stimulate the few cells in the scar tissue to restart the healing process and attracts stem cells from subcutaneous tissue nearby to help (fig. 10). The result is that the collagen matrix is remodeled to be more like normal subcutaneous tissue,[26] increasing in strength and assuming a more normal appearance. In depressed scars, the addition of a little HA may be necessary to add volume and scaffolding for new fibroblasts in the subcutaneous tissue.[27]

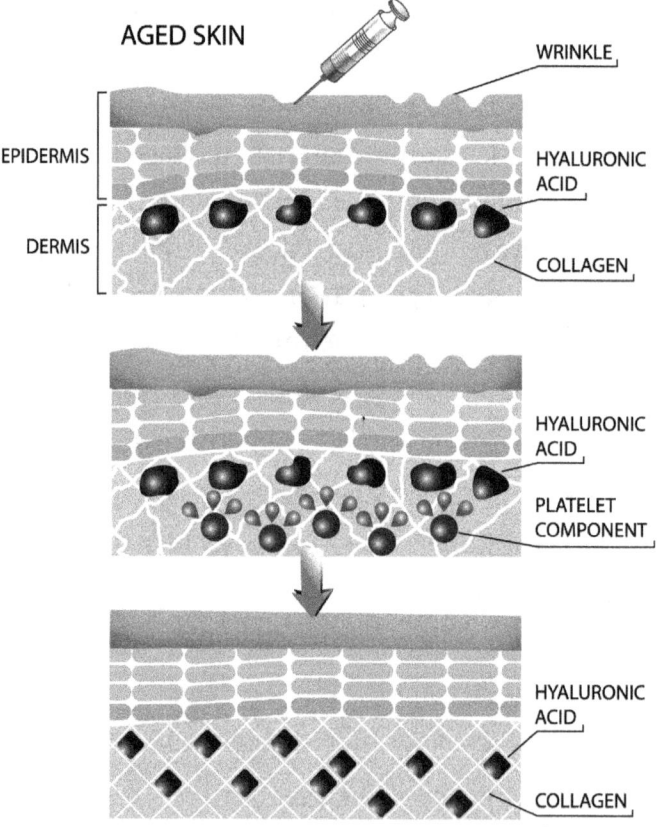

Figure 10. PRP treatment (top) releases growth factors (middle) which induces the replacement of disorganized scar tissue with new, normal skin (bottom).

Priapus Shot/Erectile Dysfunction

This technique may be both aesthetic and therapeutic. However, it is still early days and there are no published human studies. The theory is that the injection of stem cells and/or PRP into the penis will stimulate 1) tissue growth, causing the penis to lengthen and thicken, and/or 2) vascular growth, which restores the poorly responsive blood vessels in the penis that are responsible for erectile dysfunction. Preliminary private studies[28] claim an 80% success rate with the PRP procedure (dubbed the "priapus shot") in terms of aesthetics (length and girth). Success in these cases was defined as up to a one-inch increase in length and a one-inch increase in circumference.

This is obviously an area of great interest to many men and a fair amount of research is ongoing. We don't know of any randomized, double-blind, controlled human studies at present, but there is at least one pilot study underway in Florida using fat stem cells. That study is directed specifically at erectile dysfunction.[29]

Hair

Baldness is a sign of aging that affects a large portion of the male population. Women's hair tends to thin as they grow older. When it occurs at an early age it's particularly troubling in our youth-oriented society. Hair transplants have become a popular treatment, but they're frequently obvious and a very incomplete solution. Rogaine and some other drugs may also help.

This is still an area of exploration in regenerative medicine. While diseases, cancer therapy, medications, or chemicals may cause hair loss, most of the time it is caused by a combination of genetic susceptibility and hormone imbalance. The hormone in question is dihydrotestosterone (DHT), a metabolite of testosterone. As you might expect, this means that men (who have more testosterone and therefore more DHT) are more affected and they are harder to treat than women. Too much DHT makes hair follicles (the little holes in your scalp from which hair grows) shrivel up and become dormant (fig. 11). Treatment with drugs that suppress DHT, however, has been only modestly effective in many cases.

Theoretically, the injection of stem cells and/or PRP should stimulate the growth of hair follicles or reactivate the growth of hair in old ones. The best way to do this has not yet been found. Many doctors have tried injecting PRP by itself, but the results have been less than inspiring.

However, recently, Pinell has developed a technique using PRP in conjunction with vitamins and extracellular matrix material that seems to have broken the impasse. This treatment regimen has almost a 100% success rate in women with one treatment and about an 80% success rate in men with two treatments.[30]

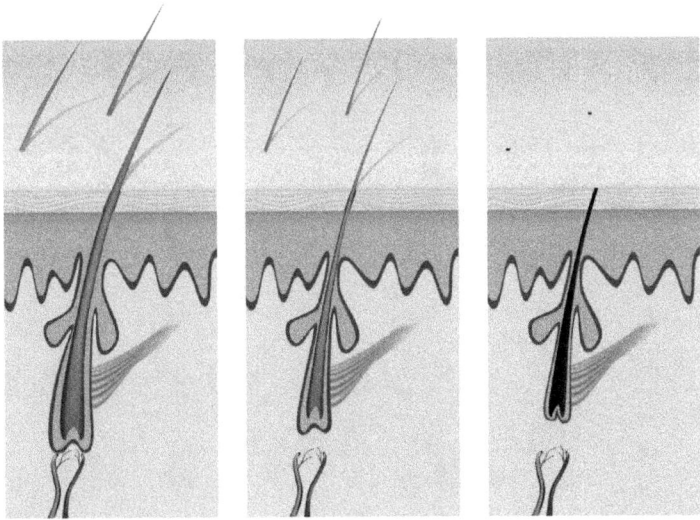

Figure 11. Most hair loss is caused by shrinking hair follicles.

PRP treatment relies a lot on there being viable hair follicles around which can be stimulated back to health. No hair follicles means no hair regrowth.

Researchers at Sanford-Burnham Medical Research Institute have gotten to the point, however, where they can produce new hair follicles in mice.[31] They take human pluripotent stem cells and induce them to differentiate into dermal papilla cells - the cells that regulate hair follicle formation. Once injected into the skin these cells cause the creation of new hair follicles with, therefore, new hair. It will be a few years before this reaches the market for humans, but chances are that even if your hair is completely gone you'll be able to grow it back.

4

Therapeutic Procedures

Prolotherapy has been around for more than seventy years, but its recent combination with PRP and stem cells has turned it into a powerful therapeutic modality.

Chronic Back Pain

Case report

Stan Mikita was a championship hockey player in the 1960s and 70s. Unfortunately, he injured his back during the 60s and suffered with chronic back pain. Matters came to a head about six weeks before the 1971–72 training camp. The pain got so bad that he couldn't even get out of bed. He had gone to the best sports medicine clinics and rehabilitation specialists without notable success.

However, he had read about prolotherapy, so he called Gustav Hemwall, MD, the world's preeminent prolotherapist at the time and made an appointment. Dr. Hemwall treated Mikita's lower back twice in three weeks – fairly aggressive treatment–because the training camp was looming. The results, to quote Mikita, "Were unbelievable! For the last eight years of my career I was completely pain free."[32]

Back pain is an extremely common, almost universal, affliction. It's said that 80 to 90% of Americans get it at one time or another in their lives. Although there are myriad causes, the underlying pathology is usually deterioration of the hundreds of ligaments and tendons in the back. This, in turn, is caused by the constant stress of gravity (we aren't entirely adapted to bipedalism yet) and the fact that almost every movement we make involves the structures of the back.

The spine has almost one-third of all the joints in the body. Each vertebra (bone in the spine) has, of course, a joint with the vertebra above and below it, with disks in between. But each vertebra also has a "spinous process" of bone that extends out the back of the vertebra and surrounds the spinal column.

Each spinous process also has four "facet" joints, two with the vertebra above and two with the vertebra below. So if you count them all up, there are 22 disk joints and 44 facet joints, a total of 66 joints, in the spine. Multiple ligaments and tendons anchor every one of those joints (fig. 12). That's a lot of places where something can go wrong.

As we age, ligaments and tendons weaken. Add sports and work injuries and the daily traumas of everyday life and eventually something is bound to give. Fortunately, when we're young the body's healing system swings into action and usually does a pretty good job of regenerating damaged tendons and ligaments. But not always. And even less so as we get older. Thus, the little (or big) insults and injuries accumulate and the tendons and ligaments just don't hold the joints as tightly as they once did. Loose joints wiggle around and stretch nerves. They allow bones to rub against each other where they normally wouldn't. The result is inflammation and pain.

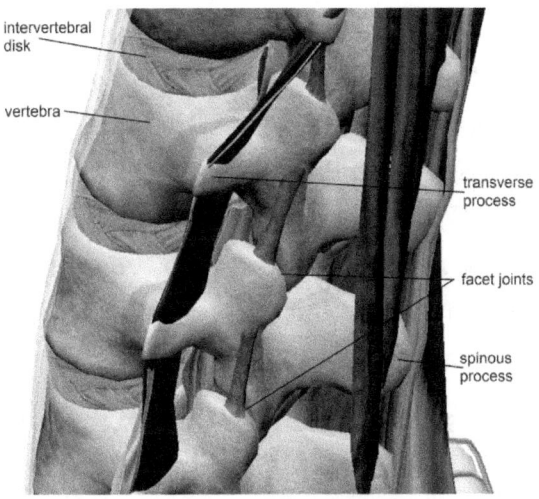

intervertebral
disk

vertebra

transverse
process

facet joints

spinous
process

Figure 12. Each bone in the spine has six joints and a host of small ligaments and tendons.

Then there are the disks. The spine consists of a stack of bones called vertebrae. In between each pair of vertebrae in the stack is an intervertebral disk, which consists of a tough outer fibrous membrane and an inner elastic core. The disk acts as a shock absorber between the vertebrae. Over a lifetime these shock absorbers get many shocks and it's not surprising that they begin to wear out. A weakness in the outer membrane can allow the inner core to bulge out, like a little balloon, and that bulge can impinge on a nerve or other structures, causing pain. In addition, the weakening and change in shape of the disk causes stresses and stretching of ligaments and tendons in the area as they try to compensate. This probably contributes more to back pain than the disk problem itself.

In fact, oddly, studies show that finding a bulging disk on an MRI scan doesn't correlate with having back pain. A retrospective study of about 5000 people's backs found that about half of them had bulging disks. Also about half had back pain, but it wasn't the same half. The back pain was evenly distributed between those with bulges and those without. This would make you suspect that a lot of back pain has nothing to do with bulging disks; and therefore, finding a bulging disk on MRI does not mean that that is the cause of the back pain.

Normally rest and some pain medication will result in a resolution of symptoms. Pain, after all, is your body's way of telling you that a joint needs to rest so that it can heal. Steroid injections can give transient relief because they decrease inflammation, but multiple injections run the risk of making the problem worse because steroids actually inhibit healing. Sometimes physical therapy, TENS, acupuncture, and exercise can help. Often chiropractic manipulation is effective too, because it realigns the joints so that they don't stretch and rub.

Nevertheless, sometimes none of these methods gives permanent relief because the underlying problem of loose ligaments and tendons remains. At this point the idea of surgery is usually introduced. Unfortunately, surgery has a poor track-record of relieving back pain. Furthermore it's expensive, risky, and there's significant recuperation and rehabilitation time.

Some researchers have concluded that as much as 90% of the half million or more disk surgeries done every year are unnecessary. Worse, only about half of the patients get even some relief of pain from back surgery and 25% may even get worse. Some 50,000 patients per year even get the official diagnosis of "failed low back surgery syndrome." It's no wonder that there is a 41% increase in the use of narcotic pain medication in people who have back surgery.

Prolotherapy, on the other hand, has a good (though not perfect) track record: it is essentially painless; is virtually risk free; takes only an hour; and is relatively inexpensive. It's hard to imagine why anyone would undergo surgery without at least trying prolotherapy first.

During a prolotherapy treatment, the doctor injects small amounts of dextrose (sugar) solution and/or PRP and/or stem cells around the joints of the back. As we explained in the prolotherapy section, this causes new healing to start in the area, with growth in size and strength of the tendons and ligaments. They tighten up the joints, which in turn reduces the stretching of nerves and the friction of bones and joints, thus reducing inflammation and the attendant pain. Also, the results are nearly permanent (normal aging still takes place) although it may take up to ten treatments to get there.

The first randomized, double-blind, controlled study of the use of prolotherapy in the treatment of back pain was published in 1987.[33] At that time it was not exactly clear how prolotherapy worked, but it was clear, from animal studies, that it induced the growth of stronger and thicker tendons and ligaments rather than just producing scar tissue.[34]

In the 1987 study, 82 patients with chronic low back pain were enrolled. 91% had difficulty sitting for any length of time; 65% had difficulty sleeping because of pain; 17% had difficulty walking; 21% had decreased sexual activity; and 4% were bedridden.

Approximately half the group received prolotherapy and the other half received placebo injections. Of the treatment group, 87% had at least a 50% reduction in pain at six-month follow up and 37% were completely pain free, compared to 10% in the control group. And remember that the "placebo" was an injection of saline solution, which may have had some therapeutic effect itself.

Since that time other studies have been done. A review in 2007[35] concluded that "when combined with spinal manipulation, exercise, and other co-interventions, prolotherapy may improve chronic low-back pain and disability." A 2009 retrospective study of 145 low back pain patients treated with prolotherapy showed that 89%

had greater than 50% pain relief.[36] In 2010 a seven-year study of 140 low-back-pain patients found that "both pain and Quality of Life scores were significantly improved at least one year after the last treatment."[37]

However, those are just the joints. The disks between the vertebrae also deteriorate with time, which leads to stress on all the joints and even to slippage of one vertebra on another. What can we do to get the disks healthy again?

There are both officially reported[38] and anecdotal reports that stem cells injected directly into the intervertebral disks will rejuvenate them. In a phase II clinical trial Mesoblast Ltd. (an Australian company that makes proprietary mesenchymal stem cells) announced that in its 100-patient study a single injection of stem cells into the disk resulted in greater disk stability, less pain, and reduced disability over a six-month period.

Researchers have found average pain reduction greater than 50% at one year. There was also a decreased need for pain medication, improvement in function, and less need for both surgical and non-surgical spine interventions in patients with moderate to severe disc-related low back pain. There are similar reported results by physicians using autologous (from the same patient on which they are used) stem cells.

While the definitive study has yet to be done, it looks like chronic low back pain, once a common and all-but-incurable disease, may become much easier to treat.

Hand Arthritis

Forty to fifty-million people in the United States live with arthritis, mostly osteoarthritis. Medical costs for it account for about 1% of gross domestic product and some $47 billion dollars in lost earnings. Since osteoarthritis increases with age the maturing baby boomer generation is at serious risk. Nearly half of them will have some type of arthritis by the age of 80. Women are more affected than men and obesity is a major risk factor.

Hand arthritis (fig. 13) is a common manifestation. Patients notice the gradual onset of stiffness, pain, and decreased range of motion in their fingers. As the disease progresses the knuckles swell and the joints become deformed. Eventually patients lose the use of their hands.

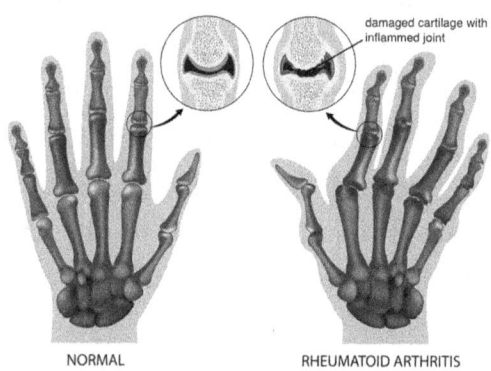

NORMAL   RHEUMATOID ARTHRITIS

Figure 13. Both cartilage in the joints and ligaments around the joints deteriorate in arthritis.

Unfortunately, there are few good clinical trials of treatments for osteoarthritis of the hand. The usual first-line treatments are pain medications, joint protection and/or splinting and local heat. Of course these are only symptomatic measures and do not do much to slow the progress of the disease.

A number of herbal remedies have been suggested, including curcumin, Boswellia, and glucosamine /chondroitin. While there are randomized controlled trials supporting the use of all three, the results are mixed for glucosamine/chondroitin. None of them, in any case, is a cure.

A last resort is arthroplasty, arthrodesis, or other surgical procedures. These frequently result in some permanent loss of function of the joint.

Standard dextrose prolotherapy of the finger joints has been around for a long time and is reported to be efficacious.[39] More recently, PRP prolotherapy of these joints is gaining popularity. The author is unaware of any reports of stem cell prolotherapy for hand arthritis.

In PRP prolotherapy the doctor draws blood and prepares PRP. He then injects a small amount into the ligament insertions on each side of the joint and a small amount into the joint itself. It takes only about 1–2 cc of PRP per joint. The treatment may have to be repeated in 4–6 weeks or even multiple times.[40]

Knees, Hips, Elbows and Shoulders

Case report

A 69-year-old gentleman presented with a rotator cuff [see fig. 14] injury of the shoulder. Two orthopedic surgeons had told him that his shoulder had deteriorated too much and that even surgery would not help. He was told to live with the chronic shoulder pain and disability.

After a thorough evaluation it was determined that he was a good candidate for prolotherapy. He received six prolotherapy treatments at three-week intervals. During the treatment period he was allowed to gradually resume his exercise regimen and after 15 weeks he was back to his usual routine of weight lifting and horseback riding. By the end of treatment he was essentially back to normal. [41]

Arthritis (from Latin, *arth* means "joint" and *itis* means "inflamed") of the large joints is a major cause of chronic pain and frequently leads to surgery. Sometimes even surgery is not appropriate as in the case report above. Nevertheless, hundreds of thousands of joint replacement surgeries are performed every year in the United States alone. These operations are expensive and risky, and may cause significant side effects, such as blood clots, infection, and allergic reactions. In fact about 3% of hip replacements have problems that are serious enough to require the intensive care unit.

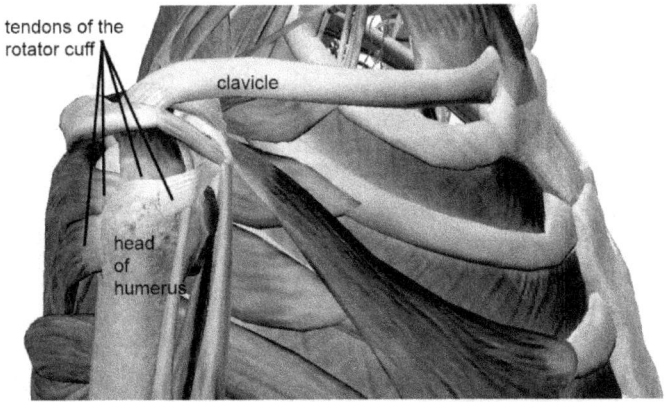

tendons of the
rotator cuff

clavicle

head
of
humerus

Figure 14. The rotator cuff is a group of tendons that insert onto the head of the humerus and rotate your arm.

The first line of treatment for arthritis is anti-inflammatory medication. If that doesn't work, the next step is usually steroid injections. Both of these treatments only take care of the symptoms and probably make the underlying disease worse. Inflammation is annoying, but it is there for a reason. It's an integral part of the body's healing mechanisms. When you suppress inflammation you also suppress healing. Therefore, while you're relieving the pain, you're also weakening the ligaments and tendons, which leads to even more joint instability and deterioration.

Eventually many patients end up in an orthopedic surgeon's office. However, surgery may not work either and it may make pain worse if it doesn't address the underlying problems.

While there are many causes of joint pain, osteoarthritis is by far the most common. It comes on insidiously, developing over many years, though the pain may come on suddenly. It doesn't show up on X-rays until it is already far progressed and the X-ray findings don't correlate with the symptoms, so somebody with normal X-rays may have severe pain, while another person with terrible looking X-rays may have no pain at all.

Even MRI scans are unreliable. A 2006 study of knee MRIs[42] showed that MRIs gave false positive findings (i.e. the MRI was interpreted as showing a problem, but on actual examination the alleged damage was not there) 65% of the time for the medial meniscus, 43% for the lateral meniscus, 47.2% for the anterior cruciate ligament, and 41.7% for cartilage disease. Frankly, much of what we think we see on joint X-rays and MRIs simply isn't really there.

Much of the pain may not come from the inside of the joint. Overuse, injuries, and daily wear and tear can gradually cause weakening and loosening of the ligaments around a joint. Then a vicious cycle may ensue in which the loose joint causes worsening osteoarthritis and the worsening arthritis causes deterioration of the joint, loosening it even more. If surgery is performed which only addresses the joint problem, but does not do anything about the ligament problem (or even makes it worse) then the treatment will not be successful. Frequently the surgeon will remove structures that the joint needs for cushion and stability. It is no surprise that long term results of these procedures include continued knee pain, knee instability, knee popping or clicking, knee weakness, worsening osteoarthritis or bone-on-bone arthritis. On top of that there are the risks of poor healing, device failure, infection, and either blood clots or bleeding. Even if everything goes well artificial joints wear out and have to be replaced every 8 to 12 years.

Fortunately, it appears that in the future many joint replacement surgeries may no longer be necessary. Prolotherapy, especially with PRP and/or stem cells, looks like it can probably handle all but the worst cases. Sometimes, as in the example above, it can take care of cases that have progressed too far for surgery.

Because prolotherapy is minimally invasive (it's only a few needle sticks), the damage done to tissues around a joint is trivial compared to the massive disruption caused by a joint replacement. These big operations necessarily involve cutting, stretching and sewing many tendons, ligaments, and muscles in the joint area. This may cause scarring or just poor healing that leaves the surrounding structures worse off than they were before.

Prolotherapy, on the other hand, involves only injecting dextrose, PRP or PRP/stem cells into the joint and the painful tendons and ligaments. While the dextrose injections may cause a little painful reaction over the first few days there is no recuperation time. The patient can go back to normal activities immediately. It doesn't even require a hospital because these injections can easily be done in a doctor's office.

We have described above how this works. Stem cells with their growth factors are attracted to the area and they initiate the normal sequence of healing events. This leads to growth, strengthening and tightening of the ligaments and tendons and to regeneration of the joint surfaces and bone. A number of studies and reports have shown regrowth of cartilage that was severely damaged.[43,44] The result is a significant reduction or even elimination of joint pain.

It's still early in the process so we don't know what the optimum prolotherapy regimen will turn out to be. Right now the procedure is unlikely to assure complete resolution with a single treatment. For advanced disease in major joints it seems more likely that three to five treatments of standard dextrose prolotherapy are necessary[45,46].

Using PRP or PRP with stem cells is likely to cut this number of treatments down significantly. One recent study[47] found that giving a single intra-articular (i.e. they gave only an injection into the knee joint rather than injecting all the surrounding ligaments and tendons as well, which would have been complete prolotherapy) treatment of PRP for knee osteoarthritis led to about a 50% improvement in six months' time, but 1) a second dose of PRP did not increase the improvement rate, and 2) results seemed to deteriorate a little bit after six months. A similar year-long study in 2013[48] found that pain, functional, and clinical scores all improved significantly at both 6 months and one year (fig. 15).

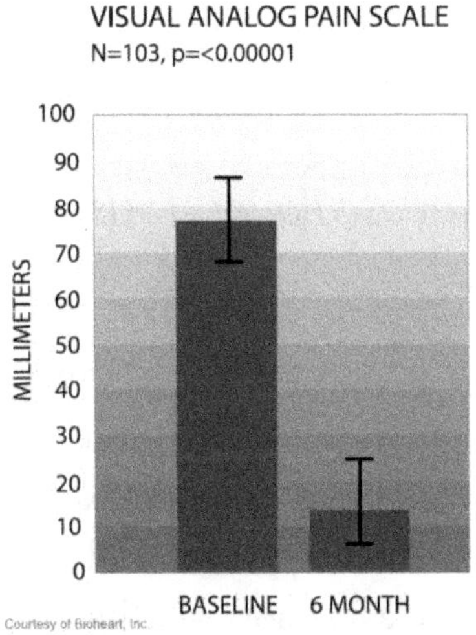

VISUAL ANALOG PAIN SCALE
N=103, p=<0.00001

Figure 15. Stem cell injection of the knee results in marked decrease in pain over a six-month period.

Of course joints other than the knee have also been studied. A small (20 patients) 2006 investigation at Stanford University[49] treated chronic tennis elbow with a single treatment of PRP prolotherapy. At eight weeks the treated patients had a 60% improvement in their pain while the controls had only 16%. Eventually, after two years, the treated group reported a 93% reduction in pain.

The largest study so far is a multicenter case series which treated 1856 joints (mostly hips and knees) in 1114 patients[50] with follow up from one to four years. The investigators gave the patients a single injection of adipose-derived stem cells in the osteoarthritic joints. They reported that twelve months after treatment 63% of the patients had a 75% improvement and 91% had at least

50% improvement. Only a handful of patients did not respond or went on to total joint replacement.

Osteonecrosis (avascular necrosis, bone infarction, aseptic necrosis)

Bone is not as solid as you might think. The outer layer is pretty dense, but inside there's the marrow with that intricate, lacy architecture, blood vessels, fat, and bone cells. Bones have three types of cells. One type breaks down bone (osteoclasts) and another type builds it up (osteoblasts). Together they constantly remodel bones to keep them strong and efficient.

Sometimes, however, things get out of balance. If the bone cells get sick or die then the bone begins to weaken and eventually it will break. Cancer and infections can cause this, but usually it is aseptic (not infectious) necrosis (cell death) – also called osteonecrosis, avascular necrosis or bone infarction.

The exact cause is not known, but it seems to be at least partially a vascular (blood vessel) problem and partially a problem of the bone stem cells and osteoblasts. There are strong associations with rheumatoid arthritis, alcohol abuse, trauma, steroids, hypertension, sickle cell anemia and at least a dozen other conditions. It can affect most any bone, but about 90% of the time it's the hip that is involved. Multiple bones may be affected (knee, shoulder, ankle, and jaw are most common after the hip).

Unfortunately osteonecrosis tends to strike a younger crowd. Most patients are in the 30-50 age range. In fact the average age is about 35-38. The USA has a few hundred thousand people with the disease and about 10-20,000 new cases appear each year. There are several treatments that may slow down or even stop the progression, but ultimately most patients end up getting a hip replacement operation. This is a tough outcome for a person in the prime of their life, especially since, as you'll recall from previous discussion, these hip prostheses need to be replaced every decade or so.

Since the 1990s a French surgeon (Hernigou[51]) has been using bone marrow stem cells to treat osteonecrosis. The technique is much simpler and safer than a hip replacement. Bone marrow is aspirated from the pelvic bone; the cells are concentrated; a needle is placed (under X-ray guidance) into the area of aseptic necrosis; the dead cells are sucked out; and the bone marrow stem cells are injected. The patient is then able to get up and go about their business. Since it is all done under local anesthesia there is no hospital stay necessary.

Dr. Hernigou's group has treated more than two thousand patients with this regimen over the last couple decades. Their success rate is about 90% with early osteonecrosis and 80% with late stage disease. This same rate of success has been duplicated by other groups in Europe. It's just starting to be used in the US where Shiple[52] has collected a case series of 20 patients in the last three years.

Fractures

Normally broken bones heal fine. But occasionally something will happen at a fracture site that will impede or prevent healing and a patient will end up with either "nonunion", i.e. a permanent fracture, or "delayed union", a fracture that is taking much longer than usual to heal. Obviously this is painful and disabling. Some bones with a poor blood supply, like the navicular bone of the wrist, are more than usually prone to this problem.

The usual treatment for this kind of problem is surgery. In the last decade more and more orthopedists have been trying PRP and stem cells as a replacement for or adjunct to surgery to try to heal fractures more quickly. This makes perfect sense because both platelets and stem cells stimulate the growth of new bone and new blood vessels. There are not very many studies, so it's too early to tell how successful this will be, but recent reports are promising.

Treatment with PRP seems to be adequate for delayed union, but not for nonunion. Two studies reported very good results when treating delayed union fractures with PRP.[53,54] Nonunion seems to require both PRP and stem cells to get the best results. Qu et al.[55] studied 72 fracture patients with fracture nonunion. Half were treated operatively and half were treated with PRP/stem cells. The former group took ten months to heal while the latter took only 5.6 months.

In any case, it's virtually always warranted to try prolotherapy before resorting to major surgery. Surgery can always be done, but it can never be undone.

Acute Injury

Traditionally physicians have waited until the normal healing processes of the body have had a chance to do their best before intervening with regenerative therapy. This usually involves watching and waiting for at least six weeks to see how an injury heals. It takes this long for tissues to go through the three phases of recovery from an injury. But there is no inherent reason why we shouldn't try a treatment that is very safe immediately to see if we can't improve the healing process, reduce down time, and get a patient pain free more quickly. Some anecdotal case reports have been published where this has been tried in professional athletes—clearly a case where time is money.

A recent announcement by Pluristem (a company that develops placenta-based stem cells) reported that in Phase I/II placebo-controlled, double-blind trials of their proprietary stem cells in patients undergoing hip replacement surgery (in which the gluteus medius muscle is damaged) the treated patients had significantly stronger and larger gluteal muscles than the placebo controls at six months post-surgery.

On the other hand, another study reported[56] that injecting PRP into the hamstring muscle of injured athletes had no effect at all on their recovery time – 42 days with or without PRP. The difference between these two studies is what the outcomes measured. So it could be that stem cell/PRP treatment may not speed up the natural healing process while it does improve the quality of recovery from an injury.

O-Shot

The O-Shot™, another invention of Dr. Charles Runels (www.oshot.info), has two main uses: relief of female urinary incontinence and enhancement of female sexual response. Stress incontinence—the involuntary leakage of urine from the bladder during physical activity such as running, jumping or during bouts of increased abdominal pressure such as sneezing or coughing—is a common occurrence in women as they get older (fig.16). Risk factors include childbirth, age, chronic cough, obesity, and smoking.

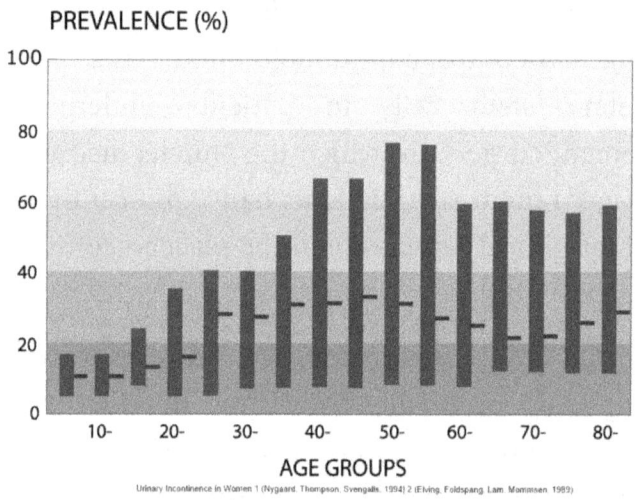

Figure 16. The prevalence of incontinence increases with age until almost 80% of women have had it.

The usual underlying cause is a loosening of the supporting tissue in the floor of the pelvis. This, in turn, can be caused by pregnancy, surgery, hormone imbalance or even by physical exercise involving frequent abrupt repeated increases in intra-abdominal pressure such as weight lifting, jogging or some forms of dancing.

The mainstays of conventional treatment are special exercises to strengthen the pelvic muscles, and failing that, surgery. Weight loss helps in overweight women.

The regenerative procedure is quite straightforward. PRP is obtained from the blood and then injected into the anterior superior vaginal wall between the vagina and the urethra (fig. 17). The idea is to increase the tissue mass and strength in this area to compensate for the local weakness.

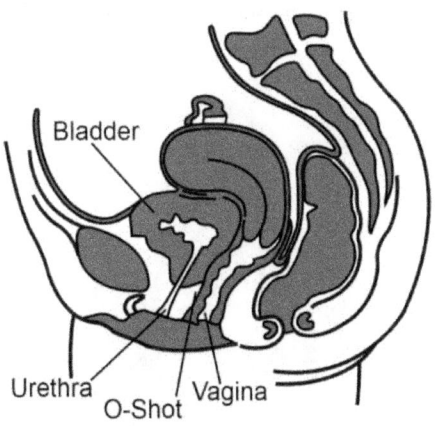

Figure 17. The O-Shot thickens the tissue between the vagina and the urethra.

As in other areas, the growth factors in the PRP attract stem cells and kickstart the process of tissue growth locally. The loose connective tissue in this area thickens mildly, but there have been no reports of scarring. This has two desirable effects: 1) the new tissue provides a more solid support for the urethra, especially near the bladder outlet, thus improving bladder sphincter control, resulting in less urinary incontinence, particularly stress incontinence. 2) The thickened wall narrows the vaginal introitus, which apparently leads to increased sensation and responsiveness during sexual intercourse.

A frequent add-on to this procedure is to inject PRP under the clitoris as well. This reportedly leads to increased clitoral sensitivity and may cause mild clitoral enlargement.

At present there have been no published studies on the effectiveness of this procedure, so all information is anecdotal.

Part III: Regenerative Treatments for Other Problems

There are two general approaches to using stem cells to regenerate organs: the *in vitro* method and the *in situ* method.

In vitro is Latin for "in glass." It refers to doing something in a test tube or flask outside the body. In regenerative medicine it refers to the technique of building an organ or tissue from stem cells in the lab and then transplanting the finished product into a patient's body. This is the most popular conception of how stem cell therapy will work.

In situ means "in place" and refers to treating an organ or tissue while it is still inside the body. In this technique stem cells are prepared and then injected into and/or around the area/organ to be treated. Examples are the prolotherapy methods discussed above.

5

Blood and Skin

Blood

Interestingly, it appears that we've been doing stem cell transplants for about 40 years and never knew it until recently. Bone marrow transplants, introduced in the 1950s, are really just transplants of blood stem cells from one person to another (fig. 18). It's an *in situ* procedure since the bone marrow is regenerated inside the patient's body.

Blood is made in your bone marrow and that is where your blood stem cells are. Fortunately, the hip bones have relatively large and easily accessible areas containing bone marrow, so that is where it is usually harvested. The doctor just inserts a needle through the outer layer of the bone into the marrow and sucks out the cells. The cells are then injected into a patient whose own blood stem cells have been destroyed by chemotherapy or radiation, usually because they have a cancer of the blood or bone marrow like leukemia or multiple myeloma. The new blood stem cells find their way to the patient's bone marrow and start to grow and divide, eventually repopulating the bone marrow with healthy blood stem cells. Bone marrow transplantation has been used more aggressively in recent years in the treatment of some other diseases like multiple sclerosis and HIV with some (but not consistent) success. A recent study from Columbia University showed that bone marrow transplant could be successful in the treatment of sickle cell disease, which is a hereditary disorder of the red blood cells.[57]

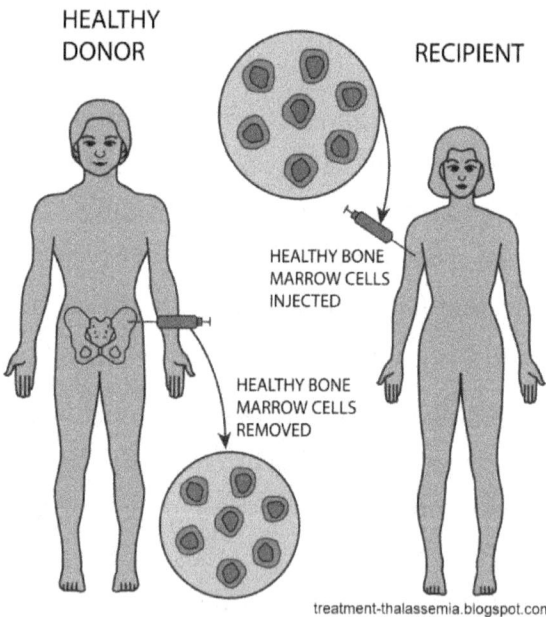

HEALTHY DONOR

RECIPIENT

HEALTHY BONE MARROW CELLS INJECTED

HEALTHY BONE MARROW CELLS REMOVED

treatment-thalassemia.blogspot.com

Figure 18. In a bone marrow transplant stem cells are taken from a donor's hip bone and injected into the recipient's vein.

This is not a benign procedure. Mortality is 10% or higher. Usually the new blood stem cells have to come from someone other than the patient and therefore there is a significant risk that the patient's body will reject the new cells (as in all such allogeneic [cells from a different patient than the one receiving them] transplants). Since the immune system (of which the blood is part) is compromised during such a transplant, infection is also a serious threat.

Not just bone marrow transplants, but blood transfusions of all kinds are a fertile field for stem cell therapies. It seems that blood shortages are always happening, and there is no way to permanently store blood. Its shelf life is only about six weeks. So far all attempts at manufacturing artificial blood have fallen short of the mark.

The first human studies on using blood cells produced from induced pluripotent stem cells are just now being planned. Cells must be reverted to iPSCs (remember them from Chapter 2?), then converted to red blood cells and finally multiplied to the needed amount. An upcoming clinical trial in Scotland will begin conservatively, with three patients who are in need of regular transfusions because they have thalassemia, a disorder of the red blood cells that causes anemia. They plan to inject the patients with about 5 mL of blood initially, and then determine whether the laboratory-made blood cells survive and behave normally once they are in the patients' bodies.

Even if it is successful this therapy still has to overcome significant hurdles in scale and the continuing problem of immunogenicity (foreign body reaction, graft vs. host disease), so we're still many years away from having a safe, usable, manufactured blood transfusion product.

The End of Antibiotics?

You're probably aware that antibiotics are becoming less "powerful." New resistant strains of bacteria are developing all the time and for some infections we've effecctively run out of anything that works.

On top of that antibiotics have side effects. They are, after all, cellular poisons that have been engineered to work well against bacterial cells and as little as possible against human cells. However, there is always overlap so there is always some effect on the human cells and that causes side effects.

So maybe we're approaching the end of the line for antibiotics. Regenerative medicine may have the solution. Our bodies have, of course, their own mechanisms for fighting infection. Your immune system recognizes foreign bacteria and sends white cells to kill them. The pus you see in some skin infections is largely white blood cells.

As we get older our immune system slows down and we become more susceptible to infections. Diabetics, cancer patients, and other people with compromised immune systems also are more vulnerable. In fact, before the age of antibiotics infections were what most people died from.

Research in this area is still in its infancy, but some animal studies have shown that it's possible to treat infections with modified white blood cells (WBCs) instead of antibiotics. Surprisingly, in one trial they used treated human WBCs on infected mice and the treated mice not only had a much lower mortality rate, but they did not suffer any immune reaction from the injected human WBC stem cells.[58]

Bonus! Stem cells may also be good fighters against viral infections that normal antibiotics can't touch. HIV (AIDS) is one such virus. The drugs used now against HIV are toxic and expensive. They can frequently halt progression of AIDS, for instance, but they can't really cure it.

However, we know that there are people who have genes that make them naturally immune to HIV. There have been a number of case reports of patients with HIV who had bone marrow transplants (for cancer) from HIV-immune donors and were essentially cured of their HIV. The theory is that HIV-immune stem cells in the transplanted bone marrow regenerated the recipient's immune system (immune system cells like white blood cells are generated in the bone marrow, just like other blood cells). With a healthy immune system HIV patients are able to fight off infections and cancer—major causes of death in HIV patients.

Nor do we need to be reliant on finding people who have natural viral immunity. A team of hematologists at the University of California have reportedly already hacked the genome of induced pluripotent stem cells (iPSCs) and produced HIV resistant white blood cells. There is much work still to be done of course, but in principal we can foresee the end of the age of antibiotics.

Skin

Skin is the easiest organized tissue to grow from stem cells. It's a simple, almost two-dimensional, tissue with only a few cell types. We already use skin grafting extensively in the treatment of burns. Adding stem cells to the transplant (just as we add stem cells to fat transplants as described in Chapter 3) is likely to produce more rapid growth and better survival of skin grafts.

Researchers at Wake Forest are starting to use 3-D printing of skin stem cells to treat burns. They scan the burn first to determine the depth of injury and then use a 3-D cell printer to fill the skin defect with the appropriate kinds of cells. This is a great improvement over standard skin grafts, which require harvesting skin from other parts of the body and then placing pieces of skin onto the burn wound.

6

Hollow Organs

After blood and skin, hollow organs, ones shaped like tubes or balloons, are the easiest to grow. They're really similar to skin except formed into a three-dimensional shape, but because of this quality they need a scaffold or mold to grow into the right configuration. The most common technique for creating scaffolding is to either make an artificial scaffold from biocompatible material or to take a cadaveric or animal organ and remove all the cells from it, leaving just the connective tissue. Stem cells are then added to the scaffold; cultured; and in time they completely populate the scaffold and differentiate to form new functional tissue.

So far we've seen this done with the trachea (fig. 19), the bladder and the esophagus, but it's only a matter of time before we see intestines, urethras, stomachs, even blood vessels. The problems with growing organs, however, are that 1) it takes a long time, maybe as long as six months, and 2) it's very expensive—in the hundreds of thousands of dollars. This method will remain in the realm of research until these issues are dealt with.

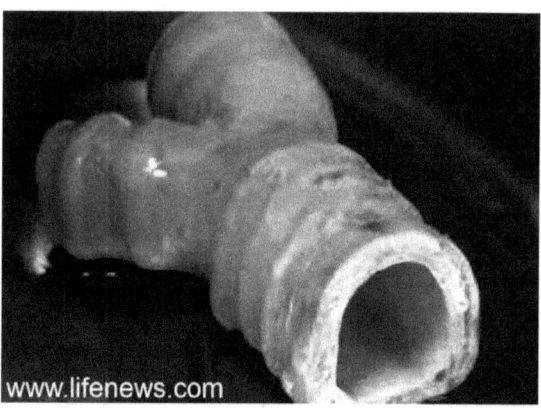

Figure 19. Tracheas grown from stem cells can be transplanted to replace ones damaged by disease, trauma or cancer.

Above we mentioned a promising new method for approaching *in vitro* stem cell transplantation: biological 3-D printing. You've probably heard of 3-D printing by now. It's a process where objects are created by having a printhead lay down layer after layer of material (plastic, metal, etc.) so that a three-dimensional object is gradually built up. Originally 3-D printers could print only one material, so you could print something that was all plastic or all metal, but not both. Now with multiple printheads laying down different materials composite objects are possible.

It turns out that you can print tissues too. You need multiple printheads, each one supplied with cells of a different tissue type. When the printer prints instead of laying down dots of ink or tiny drops of plastic it deposits individual cells in a predefined structure. Thus, if you have the appropriate types of partially differentiated stem cells and a little connective tissue glue to hold them all together you can theoretically print any organ for which you have the resources and can write the program.

This technology is in its infancy right now, but it holds promise as a way to reduce both the time and expense of creating *in vitro* organs for immediate transplant.

In the meantime *in situ* regeneration may prove to be more cost effective. Rather than grow a whole new organ and transplant it into the body to replace an old one it might work better to place stem cells in or near damaged tissue still in the body and let them use the already existent scaffolding. This is essentially what we do now in stem cell prolotherapy, where we are regenerating ligaments and tendons.

We know a lot less about trying this method on hollow organs. One of the issues is the matter of control. The scaffolding may be damaged (for instance, in a cancer) but in general we may not be able to tell. We can't control the environment in which the stem cells grow, unlike growing a cell culture outside the body, so we can't ensure that the stem cells get proper nutrition or that they get the correct signals to differentiate properly.

Peripheral Vascular Disease

Nevertheless, there is one area in which *in situ* hollow organ generation has been successfully employed – making new blood vessels. This makes perfect sense since we know that many of the growth factors found in stem cells have to do with angiogenesis (the making of new blood vessels).

Peripheral Vascular Disease (PVD, or peripheral artery occlusive disease (PAOD)) is a catch-all term for the results of a number of different diseases and processes that cause narrowing of the arteries. This usually effects the legs and results in pain or cramping, sores, cold feet, bluish skin on the legs, and decreased hair and nail growth. The current treatment is to treat the underlying cause (diabetes, smoking, high blood pressure, etc.). But frequently the disease progresses to gangrene despite treatment, eventually requiring vascular surgery and/or amputation of the limb.

These patients need new blood vessels. Stem cells can supply them. Most of the work in this area seems to be taking place in Eastern Europe and India, so we don't hear much about it in North America. But what we do hear sounds pretty good.

An open-label phase Ib trial (results announced by TotipotentRX and ThermoGenesis Corp.) was done in India over twelve months during 2013. Seventeen patients were treated with bone marrow stem cells. All the patients had critical limb ischemia (poor blood flow) and were scheduled for leg amputation before they entered the study. Remarkably at the end of the study 82% of the participants had been saved from surgery. In addition, the group had significantly reduced pain on walking, improved walking distance, and increased vasculogenesis (generation of new blood vessels) in the treated leg. Another study, of 96 patients in the Czech Republic[59], showed about a 50% reduction in major limb amputation (fig. 20).

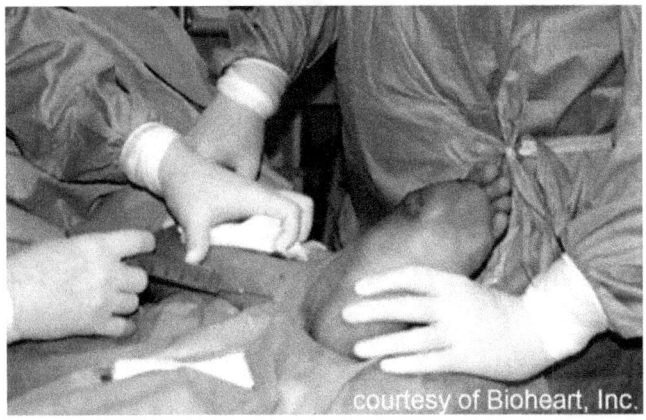

Figure 20. Stem cell therapy may prevent amputation in dying limbs.

However, the news is not all good. In 2012 a small trial (nine patients) was published in which the investigators used stem cells derived from blood (not bone marrow or adipose tissue) and them injected into the limbs of patients with critical limb ischemia. While four patients improved and one was lost to follow up, two patients had heart attacks, one died from a mesenteric thrombosis, and another from congestive heart failure.[60]

It's hard to know whether the therapy contributed to any of these deaths. But the results highlight the fact that until we have large randomized, controlled trials we really won't know the complications and their rates of occurrence.

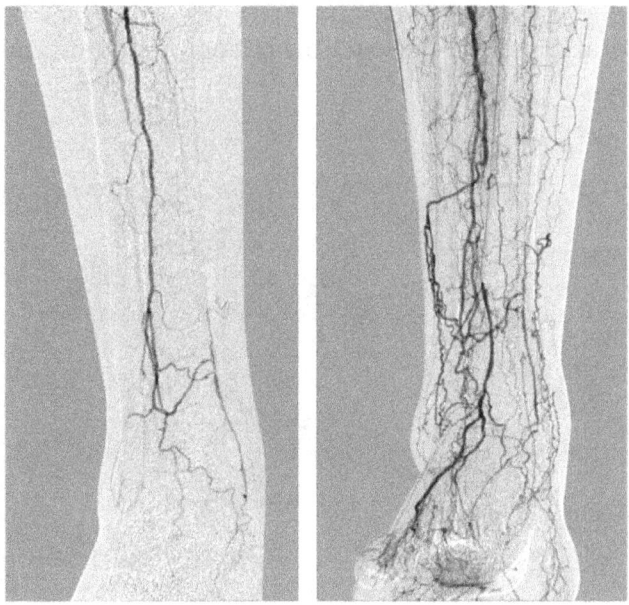

Courtesy of Bioheart, Inc.

Figure 21. An arteriogram showing leg blood flow before (left) and after stem cell treatment.

One good study comparing stem cell sources showed that it may make a significant difference where they come from.[61] Fat stem cells may be better at making new blood vessels than bone marrow stem cells and bone marrow stem cells may be better at other things. The bottom line is that the angiogenic (blood vessel forming) growth factors in stem cells seem to live up to their potential and are, in fact, able to grow new blood vessels for people with an ailing vascular system. Clinical trials on this question are underway in the USA.[62]

7

Solid Organs

These are the hardest organs to regenerate. Solid organs like the heart and the kidney have not only a complex anatomical structure, but also many different specialized cell types. Further, the architecture and the physiology of the organ frequently are interdependent, such that the cells must be organized in a particular way in order for the organ to work properly. It wouldn't work, for instance, if the cells that produce urine in the kidney were located anywhere other than right next to the ducts that collect urine.

Heart

Regenerative therapy of the heart is being done both *in situ* and *in vitro*. The heart, believe it or not, is a relatively simple organ. It's mostly muscle and connective tissue but has some specialized cells for electrical conduction and to produce a heartbeat. When someone has a heart attack one of the blood vessels supplying the heart muscle is plugged up and blood can't get to the muscle beyond to supply it with oxygen and nutrients. That muscle dies unless the blood supply is restored in a hurry (fig. 22).

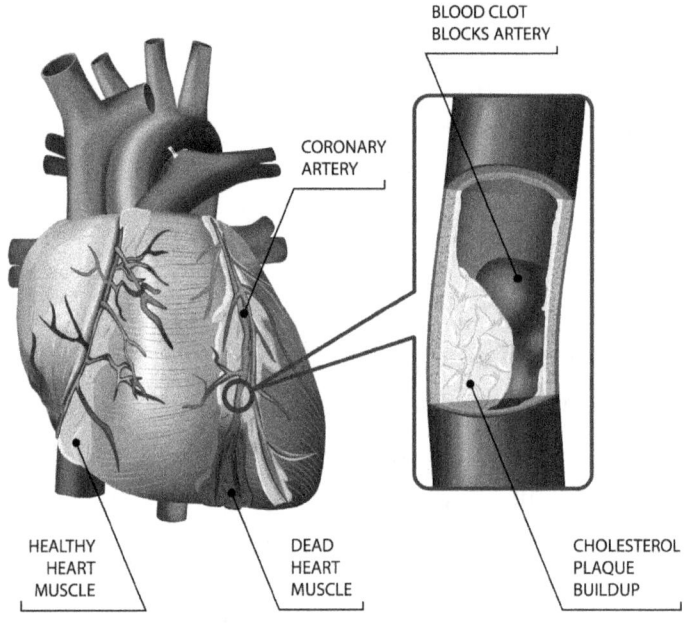

Figure 22. In a heart attack the heart muscle partly dies and is weakened. Congestive heart failure can result.

If the patient survives the heart attack the dead muscle turns into a scar. It doesn't contribute to heart contractions anymore and this makes the heart pump blood less efficiently. This can lead to congestive heart failure in which the heart's inefficiency causes fluid to build up in the lungs. Eventually this can be fatal.

There are good drugs for heart failure, but obviously they are just temporizing measures. They don't build back the missing muscle. The only "cure" right now is a new heart—a heart transplant.

But available hearts for transplant are scarce. This is where the *in vitro* method is being researched. If we only had new hearts readily available, then everybody who needed one could get one. So why not just grow new hearts and keep them in stock?

This has been done in animal studies and it's not as hard as you might think. The critical requirement is a scaffold on which to put the stem cells so that they can grow into a heart. In a living heart the connective tissue performs the task of holding all the cells in the right place, so the easiest way to get a scaffold is to take a cadaver heart and remove all the cells. This is not so difficult with the right kind of detergent solution and what you are left with is a spongy kind of mass in the shape of a heart.

Then comes the hard part. How do you tell the undifferentiated stem cells what kind of heart cells they need to turn into in different parts of the heart? Fortunately for us it appears that much of this information is already contained in the connective tissue. If we just populate the scaffolding with stem cells the connective tissue matrix seems to tell the stem cells a lot about where to go and what to do.

Of course it's not quite that simple. Most of the details still need to be worked out. However you get the idea—growing a new heart has progressed way beyond the theoretical stage. And we haven't even mentioned how 3-D printing might speed this up.

The *in situ* method is much easier. Why use a scaffold outside the body for the stem cells when there is a perfectly good one already in the patient's body? Just add stem cells.

In the *in situ* method stem cells are prepared and then injected directly into the heart muscle/scar or into the coronary arteries (the blood vessels that supply the heart muscle) through a long catheter that is threaded up into the heart from the groin through a major blood vessel. Under X-ray guidance the physician can see exactly where he is injecting the cells to make sure that he places them where they will do the most good (fig. 23).

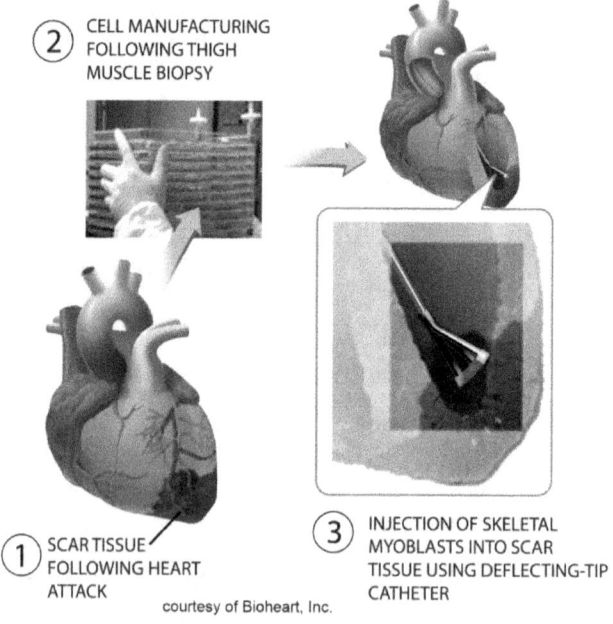

② CELL MANUFACTURING FOLLOWING THIGH MUSCLE BIOPSY

① SCAR TISSUE FOLLOWING HEART ATTACK

③ INJECTION OF SKELETAL MYOBLASTS INTO SCAR TISSUE USING DEFLECTING-TIP CATHETER

courtesy of Bioheart, Inc.

Figure 23. Stem cell injections restore heart muscle.

Once in place the stem cells do their job under the influence of the surrounding cells and connective tissue. They secrete their growth factors and cytokines. They replicate and build new muscle and connective tissue. They create new blood vessels to supply the new muscle.

When they are done the patients have a more muscular heart that can beat harder and pump better. Fluid in the lungs dissipates and they are able to breathe more easily and exert themselves more (figs. 24,25). Quality of life is substantially improved.

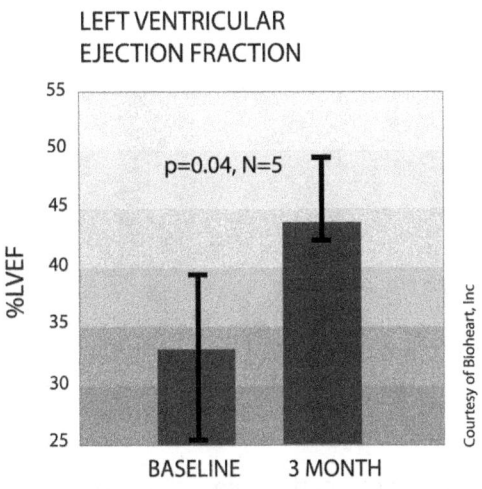

Figure 24. The amount of blood the heart pumps can more than double after stem cell treatment.

This method of heart regeneration is already in clinical trials. Several small studies have been done and published[63]. Reserchers in the United Kingdom have organized a study involving 3,000 patients in 11 European countries that hopefully will show definitively whether stem cell treatments can cut the death rates and repair damaged tissue after a person has a heart attack. Patients who suffer heart attacks will undergo the normal procedure of having a stent placed to keep their arteries open, but also will be injected with their own bone marrow stem cells. Because of the large data set, this trial should give a much clearer answer whether or not stem cells effectively heal cardiac tissue. We'll know the answer in about 2019.

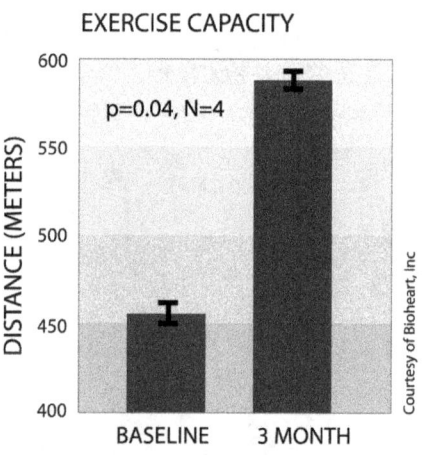

Figure 25. The distance a patient can walk can quadruple when heart muscle is restored with stem cells.

Pancreas

There is a worldwide epidemic of diabetes going on right now so there is intense interest in finding ways to ameliorate or cure these diseases. We say disease"s" because there are two different kinds of diabetes. They both affect the pancreas, but their pathological mechanisms are entirely different. It's unlikely that a single cure will be found that works for both types.

Researchers have been working on pancreas transplants since your author was in medical school (a long, long time ago), but it's only recently that substantial progress has been made. The pancreas, like other solid organs, is a very complicated structure and performs many different tasks for the body. It's not very easy just to transplant or grow a new one (fig. 26).

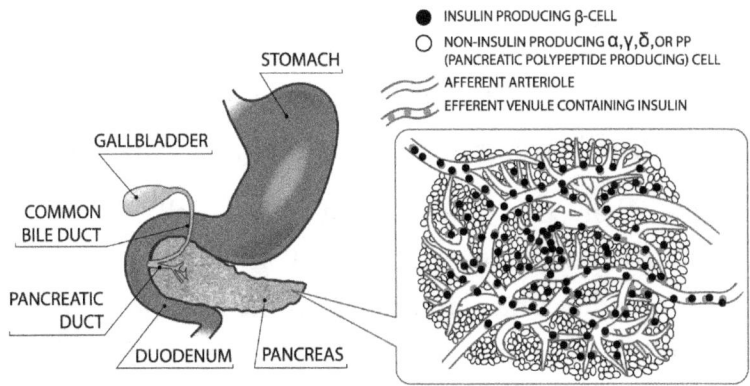

Figure 26. The pancreas sits right under the stomach and secretes digestive enzymes into the bowel and insulin and other hormones into the blood.

In both types of diabetes the end result is that the beta cells of the pancreas "burn out" and don't produce enough (or any) insulin any more. Since insulin is essential for getting energy (as glucose) into cells we need either to replace the insulin or replace the cells that make insulin to keep diabetics alive.

Fortunately there have been many promising studies lately on this front. The one that caught our eye today was typical:

A company in Australia reported a phase II randomized, single-blind, placebo-controlled dose-escalation study in which they injected 61 human type 2 diabetics with a single intravenous infusion of the company's proprietary mesenchymal stem cells. They watched them for twelve weeks and followed their hemoglobin A1c levels (HbA1c is a measure of how high their blood glucose levels were over that time). At the highest dose of stem cells HbA1c levels were significantly reduced, indicating that the injected stem cells had indeed at least partially restored the function of the pancreas.

Note that this method of stem cell therapy is particularly advantageous in that it requires only IV access. You don't have to grow a whole new pancreas and you don't have to undergo a transplant operation. If these stem cells or any of their similar competitors make it through phase III trials in the next few years we will see a revolution in the way that diabetes is treated.

In a related area, however, there already is good evidence for clinical use of stem cells. Type 2 diabetes is frequently complicated by peripheral neuropathy (damage to small nerves in the hands and feet, which results in pain and/or numbness) and peripheral arterial occlusive disease (damage to the blood vessels of the arms and legs, resulting in ulcers and eventually, gangrene). Since blood vessel growth factors are a significant component of the apparatus of stem cells logically you would think that they might help repair this damage. Indeed, clinical trials and case reports of using mesenchymal stem cells have shown that this is a viable treatment alternative, especially for non-healing diabetic foot ulcers.[64] See also the discussion above about peripheral vascular disease.

Kidney

One of the main causes of kidney disease is diabetes, so just as there is an epidemic of diabetes worldwide, there is a sub-epidemic of renal failure. Unfortunately there is no treatment for this problem. Although there are some drugs and supplements that may slow down the progression or help stabilize the disease, the mainstays of treatment are control of the diabetes and control of high blood pressure. None of these things, however, results in a cure. The best that can be hoped for is to slow the steady deterioration of kidney function and stave off dialysis or kidney transplant for as long as possible.

Ideally there would be a new kidney waiting for each patient who deteriorated to the state of needing dialysis. Then the patient would just get a kidney transplant and be almost as good as new. But as usual there are a few problems.

1. There are not enough transplant kidneys to go around, so there is a waiting list. While waiting you may have to go on dialysis. In some countries the situation is such that if you are beyond a certain age they won't even put you on the waiting list because they deem the benefit you will obtain from a new kidney is less than what a younger patient would get. In that case you have to go find your own kidney donor.

2. Under the current state of the art even a kidney transplant is no panacea. It's still someone else's kidney and there is the risk of rejection and the side effects of the drugs you have to take to minimize that risk.

Dialysis has its own set of complications. It doesn't do nearly as good a job as a real kidney does and there are significant potential complications and side effects. The average life expectancy of a patient once they have to go on dialysis is about five years.

Big problem = big opportunity. This disease is the ideal candidate for stem cell regenerative medicine. But it's not easy. The kidney is one of the most complex organs in the human body. It is not only anatomically complex, but also a physiological powerhouse with many different cell types and multiple different functions. It controls hydration of the body, balances the blood electrolytes, affects blood pressure, secretes a variety of hormones and, of course, eliminates bodily wastes.

We used to think that once the kidney developed it pretty much stayed the same throughout adult life and had limited, if any, regenerative and repair capabilities. Kidney stem cells seemed pretty rare and not all that active. Recent research, however, has contradicted that view to some extent. Researchers at Stanford and Tel Aviv's Sheba Medical Center have found that, at least in mice, the kidney rejuvenates itself, remodels and continues to generate specialized kidney cells all the time. The complication is that it seems there is not just one "kidney stem cell." Each functional part of the kidney appears to have its own dedicated type of stem cell. Nevertheless, the investigators found that there does seem to be a common controlling pathway and the principal investigator opined that "We may be able to turn on the pathway to generate new kidney-forming cells."[65]

Both *in situ* and *in vitro* methods of regeneration are being researched and tested for kidney disease. The *in situ* method is much simpler and thus has a head start. There are clinical trials already in progress where autologous stem cells are being harvested and injected into the kidney through a catheter threaded through the main arteries of the body. It's something of a long shot, but we'll be very lucky if this treatment or some variation of it (iPSCs, or specially treated stem cells, for instance) works because the procedure is relatively simple and inexpensive.

In vitro kidney regeneration is slower in coming because of the aforementioned complexity of the organ. As of this writing researchers from Brigham and Women's

Hospital in Boston have successfully coaxed stem cells to become kidney tubular cells. The researchers discovered a cocktail of chemicals which, when added to stem cells in a precise order, causes them to turn off genes found in embryonic stem cells and turn on genes found in kidney cells, in the same order that they turn on during embryonic kidney development.

At the same time a Japanese research team from Kumamoto University has successfully created three-dimensional kidney parts from human iPSCs. The team succeeded in creating glomeruli, which filter out waste products from blood, and renal tubules, which reabsorb substances essential for the human body. The reproduced tissues, about two millimeters long, produced kidney-specific proteins but no urine.

These are steps in the right direction but it seems it will be a matter of some time before we have "off the shelf" kidneys available for transplantation when needed.

Lung

The lung isn't exactly a "solid" organ, but it is definitely quite complicated. Through 3D printing and cell cloning, now more than ever, it is possible to imagine growing "replacement parts" for the human body. The latest of these compelling stories involves the creation of human lungs by scientists in a lab at the University of Texas Medical Branch. This is one of the most impressive steps yet toward making regenerative medicine a reality—

which will eventually lead to practical options for those in need of a lung transplant.

Dr. Joan Nichols, a researcher at the UTMB, characterized it best by saying, "It's so darn cool. It's been science fiction and we're moving into science fact," according to a CNN report.

It still remains to be seen if the lungs will actually work inside a real person. However, if they turn out to be functional, being able to grow lungs and other organs in the lab would help to clear the long backlogs of patients waiting for transplants. In the case of lung transplants, there are currently about 1,600 people waiting for a new set of lungs.

The researchers at UTMB developed the process of crafting the lungs with donated lungs that were too damaged to be used in a transplant, but were intact enough to be used in the experiment. The researchers stripped away virtually everything from one of the lungs except for a remaining scaffolding of collagen and elastin. They then added cells from another lung and immersed the lung frame into a chamber filled with cell-growing nutrients. After just four weeks, a fully lab-engineered lung had grown from the scaffold and cells. They were then able to repeat the process, and craft a second lung the same way.

Researchers believe that while the lung-growing experiment worked surprisingly well, the biotechnology is not quite ready for prime time. In fact, they anticipate that it could be another 12 years before it will be possible to successfully implant lab-crafted lungs into humans. The first step will be to try out the lungs on pigs.

However where *in vitro* solutions may be difficult, *in situ* solutions may be easier. This is because when you inject any materials (like stem cells) into any vein in the body the second organ they hit is the lung. After passing through the right side of the heart all blood is filtered by the lungs. The red blood cells have to pass through tiny capillaries in this organ to release their carbon dioxide and pick up a fresh supply of oxygen. Since stem cells are attracted to damaged tissue the normal circulatory function makes it quite simple to deliver stem cells to the area of maximum utility in patients with lung disease.

Asthma and emphysema (COPD, chronic obstructive pulmonary disease) are pretty common lung diseases. Asthma is generally a disease of the young, while emphysema is a disease of the old, mostly smokers.

R. D. was a 66-year-old male with severe COPD. He had been a heavy smoker and lived and worked in an area of significant air pollution. He was diagnosed with COPD many years before seeking stem cell treatment. Despite stopping smoking and trying all that conventional medicine could offer his disease progressed to the point where he was almost bedridden and required constant oxygen therapy. He was told he had only two months left to live and was in line for a lung transplant. However, his daughter was getting married in eight months and he desperately wanted to be able to attend her wedding.

On initial evaluation he was completely dependent on supplemental oxygen and could walk only about 25 meters. After a complete workup Mr. D. was given an intravenous dose of adipose-derived stem cells. Over the next six months his lung function gradually improved. He was able to get off oxygen and at nine months (the wedding was delayed) he was able to walk his daughter down the aisle and dance with her at her wedding—without oxygen.

At one year he was given another dose of stem cells and continued to improve. He was able to go back to work. Unfortunately he eventually overdid it and died of a heart attack two and a half years after his initial treatment.[66]

In COPD chronic irritation causes inflammation in the lungs that in turn leads to breakdown of lung tissue and poor airflow (fig. 27). The most obvious symptom is shortness of breath.

Fortunately COPD can usually be prevented from worsening and even made to regress somewhat by removing the irritants (smoking, air pollution, etc.). But this doesn't work for everybody and in some cases the disease progresses to the point where only a lung transplant can help. Even if the disease progression can be halted it will mean that some patients will still be confined to chairs or bed and need a constant oxygen supply.

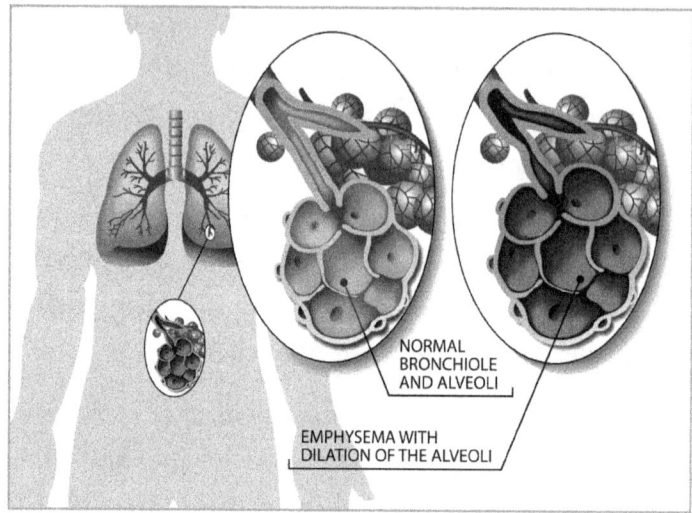

NORMAL
BRONCHIOLE
AND ALVEOLI

EMPHYSEMA WITH
DILATION OF THE ALVEOLI

Figure 27. In COPD lung tissue is gradually destroyed.

We should be able to do something about this with stem cells. Such treatments have been available in Europe for quite a few years now, but we haven't seen any published results of trials. In the United States there have been some case reports of successful treatment (fig. 28), but the clinical trials are just now getting started. It is to be hoped that we'll hear some good news in a couple years.

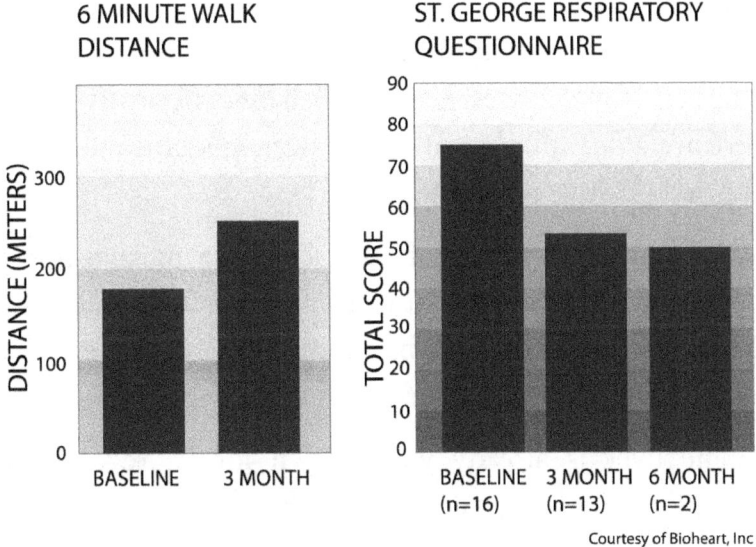

6 MINUTE WALK DISTANCE

ST. GEORGE RESPIRATORY QUESTIONNAIRE

Courtesy of Bioheart, Inc

Figure 28. After stem cell treatment the distance a COPD patient could walk doubled and breathing difficulty decreased.

Not much has been done in the way of studies of stem cell treatment of asthma. A recent review[67] concluded that some large multicenter clinical trials were needed, but even a few small studies to point us in the right direction would be welcomed.

Liver

There is a great interest in finding a cure for chronic liver disease because of the limited supply of livers available for transplant and the lack of efficacy of current treatments. Animal studies have been promising and have prompted dozens of clinical trials. As of this writing,

103

however, there have been no really good, large, randomized, double-blind controlled studies of the use of stem cells for diseases like cirrhosis and hepatitis C. But there are a fair number of minor human studies that have reported positive results.[68]

As with other trials of stem cells the mechanism of action remains unclear. But it seems that actual replication of the stem cells may not be as important as the effect of the stem cells on their environment.

The liver is already well known for its regenerative abilities. It can regrow even after a 75% loss. Recent research has shown that there may be a couple of reasons for this. The prevailing theory is that the liver just has more stem cells than most organs. However, recent findings suggest that mature liver cells easily dedifferentiate back into liver progenitor cells. That is, mature liver cells can regress to a previous stem-cell state and start duplicating to grow more liver cells. If this finding is confirmed, it means that almost all liver cells are potential stem cells and it should be relatively easy to induce or create autologous liver grafts.

Nervous system

The brain and nervous system form the most complex component of the human body. Thus we can expect it will probably be the last area in which regenerative therapies take hold.

Migraine Headache

While rarely life-threatening, migraine headaches are a serious and relatively common cause of disability, affecting about 2% of the population—mostly women. The exact cause is still unknown and the current treatments are all palliative rather than curative.

You might think migraines would be an unlikely candidate for stem cell therapy. After all, there is no known tissue defect or particular cellular dysfunction that we can hold responsible for them. Nor is there a specific anatomical location associated with them. Rather the pathology seems to be a complex mix of genetic predisposition, inflammation, neuronal excitation/inhibition, and changes in local blood flow.

Nevertheless, the involvement of inflammation has prompted some researchers to try stem cell treatment (stem cells have well known anti-inflammatory activity) on chronic migraines. The mechanism of action is, of course, completely unknown. But a case series published last year (2014) from Australia reported four cases in which each patient had significant long-term (18 months) improvement in symptoms after an intravenous injection of adipose-derived stem cells.[69]

This is only four cases, so obviously much more study is needed, but it certainly gives us an indication that a relatively simple "cure" for migraines might be close at hand.

CVA (cerebrovascular accident, or stroke)

Stroke is second only to heart disease as a cause of death worldwide, with over five million deaths per year. It is the number one cause of adult disability. There have been some advances in acute care and secondary preventive strategies, but these have barely had an impact on the overall morbidity and mortality.

Nevertheless, as I write, the news media are trumpeting the treatment of Gordie Howe, a famous championship hockey player, with a new stem cell treatment by Stemedica. Mr. Howe was brought to the hospital (in Tijuana, Mexico) by his family (including his son, an experienced MD of 30 years) barely able to talk or eat and unable to walk. He had suffered a severe stroke earlier in the year and was deteriorating—reportedly at death's doorstep. They expected he wouldn't last more than a month. A few days later after treatment with neural and mesenchymal stem cells he walked out under his own power and has since resumed a fairly normal life—for an 87 year old.

There have been quite a few phase I and phase II human studies using stem cells in the treatment of stroke. These have used various types of stem cells and different delivery methods (mostly intravenously and intra-arterially), but have generally demonstrated the safety and feasibility of treatment of both acute and chronic stroke. While none of the trials has directly addressed the efficacy of such treatment (this will come in phase III trials), there has been a general trend toward better outcomes in patients in the phase I and II studies.

Alzheimer's Disease

Alzheimer's disease is the world's most widespread degenerative neurological disease. Over five million Americans live with it, and one in three senior citizens will die from it or a similar disease. Memory loss is the most common symptom of Alzheimer's, but behavioral manifestations—depression, loss of inhibition, delusions, agitation, anxiety, and aggression—can be even more challenging.

Alzheimer's disease is caused by loss of neurons in the brain. The full mechanism isn't yet understood and current drug therapies are only modestly helpful at best.

Considering the scope and seriousness of Alzheimer's, however, there is a lot of current research looking for new ways to treat it. One promising avenue was recently described in *Behavioural Brain Research*.[70] In the study, Israeli researchers induced stem cell proliferation in the part of the brain of Alzheimer-diseased mice that controls behavior and found that they were able to get an increase in the number of normal neurons in the area. This caused the Alzheimer's mice to revert to normal behavior from their previous uninhibited Alzheimer-like behavior.

In another recent animal study Stemedica International S.A. announced the first results of a trial of intravenous administration of their proprietary allogeneic, human, ischemia-tolerant mesenchymal stem cells (itMSCs) in a preclinical animal model of Alzheimer's disease. They showed a greater than 30 percent decrease in amyloid beta (Abeta, one of the hallmarks of Alzheimer's disease) plaques in the brain of transgenic animals treated with Stemedica itMSCs compared to the control group that was treated with lactated Ringer's solution (a benign, isotonic IV solution).

Parkinson's Disease

We're still mostly at the primate stage of research in applying stem cells to Parkinson's disease. Among other things, parkinsonian patients have uncontrollable tremors, and their body movements slow down to the point that they can become immobile. Parkinson's afflicts more than a million Americans.

The disease is caused by the degeneration and death of cells producing a certain neurotransmitter molecule: dopamine. However it affects a number of other cell types in the brain as well. It's noteworthy that in one early mouse study injecting astrocyte (a different kind of brain cell) stem cells into the mouse brain helped to heal all the multiple types of neurological damage caused by Parkinson's disease, providing an overall benefit that has not been achieved in other approaches.[71]

Dr. Ruslan Semechkin, chief scientific officer of International Stem Cell Corp., recently presented results from experiments on African green monkeys with induced

Parkinson's disease to the American Academy of Neurology. Semechkin had induced Parkinson's in the monkeys and then injected human neural stem cells into their midbrains.

The idea was that the stem cells would reproduce in the monkey brains and begin producing dopamine, thus reversing the debilitating tremors. The experiment was successful and enabled, for instance, a monkey that had barely been able to hold a banana to peel and eat one as if he had no disability at all.

The most dramatic work so far, however, is from Peru. In 2010 a group there reported a case series of three severely disabled parkinsonian patients in whom they had injected bone marrow stem cells directly into their carotid artery (the big blood vessel that supplies the brain). The patients underwent a marked regression of many of their symptoms. You can see the before and after videos at www.faim.org/stemcell /brazziniinstituteasctvideos.html.

This and the work mentioned above on Alzheimer's disease implies that neurological disease can be improved by new stem cells in particular areas of the brain and that this technique may be applicable to many neurodegenerative diseases.

Amyotrophic Lateral Sclerosis (ALS, Lou Gehrig's disease)

Amyotrophic lateral sclerosis (ALS) is another neurodegenerative disorder, most widely known today for its debilitating effect on the life of famous British physicist Stephen Hawking. As with Alzheimer's disease the real underlying cause is not well understood, but it causes progressive degeneration of motor neurons in the cortex, brainstem and spinal cord, which leads to paralysis, inability to breathe and death within an average of three to five years from disease onset. No drugs are effective.

Recently stem cell therapy has emerged as a potential new way to treat ALS. While motor neuron replacement remains a focus of some studies trying to treat ALS with stem cells, there is more rationale for using stem cells as support cells for dying motor neurons because these neurons are already connected to the muscle.[72]

Researchers at the Mayo Clinic are working on a clinical trial now in which they take fat stem cells; culture them; and select stem cells that produce growth factors that will protect nerve cells from death and damage. These cells are cultured further to produce billions of the specialized stem cells, which are then injected into the patient's spinal fluid. The hope is that the nerve-protecting factors will diffuse into the spinal column and prevent or slow further progression of ALS.

On another front, Israel's Brainstorm Cell Therapeutics has completed a phase IIa trial of their proprietary stem cell preparation in ALS patients with promising results. After a single dose they observed meaningful slowing of disease progression and even regression in some cases. They're now testing a multi-dose strategy and have been designated a "fast-track" product by the FDA.

Multiple Sclerosis (MS)

MS is yet another neurological degenerative disease with unclear origin and no cure. In this case the proximate cause is the degeneration of the myelin sheath of nerve fibers (which is similar to the insulation on electrical wiring [fig. 29]). This causes the nerve signaling to malfunction and results in a wide variety of symptoms including difficulty walking, impaired vision, fatigue and pain.

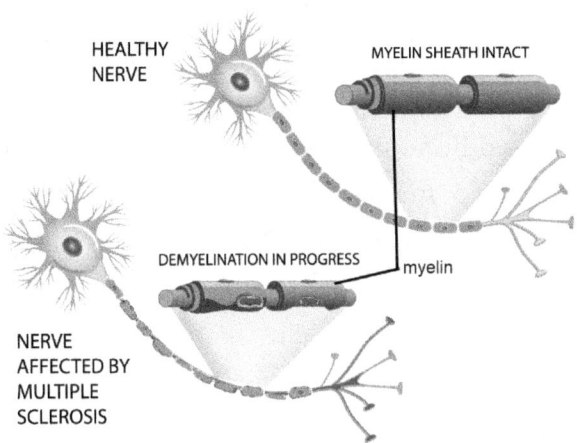

Figure 29. MS is caused by degeneration of the sheath around nerve fibers.

At the mouse stage of research recent work at the University of Utah Health Sciences Center looks promising. The investigators there induced an MS-like state in mice (which partially paralyzed them) and then injected human stem cells into their spines. By eight days there was no sign of the stem cells, but within two weeks the mice were walking and running normally. At six months they were still normal.[73]

This is another example of *in situ* stem cell therapy in which it seems the stem cells themselves are just the carriers of important growth and healing factors. It's not necessary for them to divide or grow in order for the therapy to work.

About 14 clinical trials have been registered for treatment of MS with stem cells and two have been published. One phase I/II trial from Israel used autologous stem cells injected intravenously and intrathecally (into the spinal canal). They reported no major adverse effects and some modest clinical improvement. A phase IIa study in the UK used bone marrow stem cells intravenously and also reported no major adverse events and mild clinical improvement. In a US case series in 2009, three patients given IV and intrathecal stem cells showed marked improvement.[74]

Spinal Cord Injury

Each year there are more than 10,000 new spinal cord injuries (SCI) in the United States alone. In a recent survey done by the Christopher & Dana Reeve Foundation, there were approximately 840,000 people living with chronic SCI (patients in whom paralysis persists and becomes permanent). The National Spinal Cord Injury Association says that 85% of SCI patients who survive the first 24 hours are still alive 10 years later, so this is a long-term problem.

Several studies have shown the effectiveness of stem cell transplants in spinal cord injury in rats.[75,76] At least two companies, NeuralStem and Stem Cells, Inc., are now conducting phase I human trials to establish safety of their proprietary stem cell preparations in treatment of SCI.

A third company, Asterias Biotherapeutics, has just announced the results of its phase I study in which five patients were enrolled for five years. They used derivatives of human embryonic stem cells and injected them directly into the spinal cord near the site of the injury. The researchers also lightly immunosuppressed the patients for 60 days afterwards. No significant problems were observed in the five years since treatment. Unfortunately, no significant clinical improvement was noted either. Nevertheless, phase I trials are only designed to test safety, not efficacy, and the dose of stem cells given was rather low, so the clinical results should not be given too much weight. Asterias is now starting a phase I/II dose escalation trial in cervical spinal cord injuries.

A number of researchers are using olfactory bulb (a part of the brain near the upper inner part of the nasal cavity) stem cells to try to repair SCI. These cells seem to have special properties that facilitate the regrowth of nerves through scar tissue that forms after an injury. A recently reported case had surgeons at the Wroclaw

University Hospital in Poland implanting the olfactory bulb stem cells in the spine of a young man who had his spinal cord severed in a knife fight in 2010. It has taken about two years, but the patient (who was completely paralyzed below the waist) has regained his ability to walk with the help of a walker and to drive a car.

Interestingly, among the eleven registered clinical trials of stem cells in spinal cord injuries two are phase III trials from China and Korea. There is good reason to hope that these studies will show return of movement and sensation in patients. We should see some preliminary announcements this year and more published studies in the next year or two.

Autism

The CDC estimates that 1% of the US population has autism spectrum disorder. People with autism have difficulty with language and social interaction. It's a complicated disease that has both genetic and environmental components. There is no cure.

Research in autism offers promising examples of the indirect use of stem cells to combat disease. One of the helpful properties of stem cells is that they allow us to try out drugs on human cells without putting humans at risk. Animals are traditionally used to test drugs, but of course their DNA is different from human DNA and their responses to drugs are frequently not the same as human responses. Testing using human stem cells is therefore more likely to accelerate the development of new drugs. This applies to all drugs, not just ones used for Autism.

Researchers at University of California at San Diego found that neurons (brain cells) from autistic patients were different from normal neurons, but these cells became more normal when they were cultured with normal astrocytes (another kind of brain cell). This implies that something is lacking from autistic astrocytes that can reverse the differences in autistic neurons. Theoretically the isolation of these factors could lead to effective drugs to treat autism. Even better, many potential drugs can be tested on neurons derived from autistic stem cells to determine which work and which don't. This is much faster than animal studies and much safer than human studies.

Other research has shown that autistic children have abnormalities of their immune system cells. This has led researchers to theorize that if such cells could be replaced (by stem cells) it would improve the disease. Only a single phase I trial has been completed at this time. It used umbilical cord stem cells and monocytes (another kind of white blood cell) and reported no major adverse events and some clinical improvement.[77]

Eyes

Macular Degeneration

Age-related macular degeneration (AMD) is a degenerative disease of the eyes that results in gradual central visual loss (fig. 30). It affects about ten million people in the United States, with onset around the ages of 50 or 60, and comes in two types, wet and dry. The wet version is more severe, but the dry version is more common—about 85% of cases. There is no cure for either type.

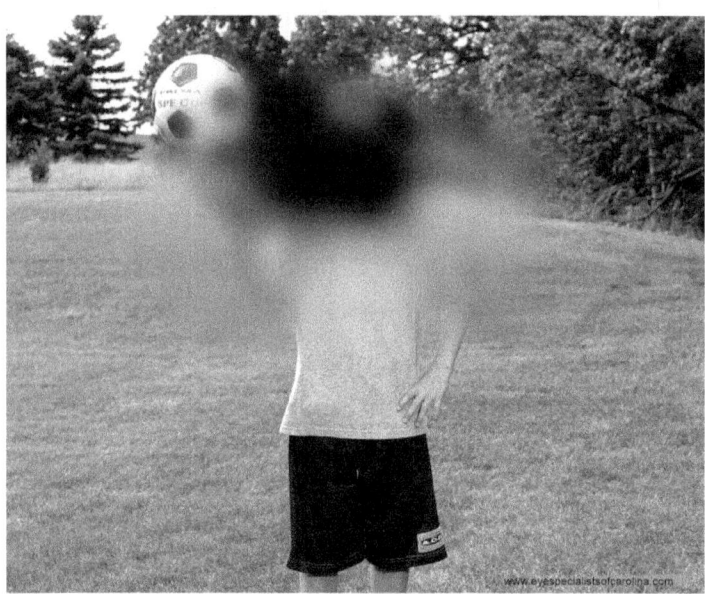

Figure 30. In macular degeneration people lose their central vision. This is what their view looks like.

StemCells Inc. is in the middle of an eight-patient phase I/II trial for advanced dry age-related macular degeneration. Its scientists are injecting one million of their proprietary stem cells directly behind the eyeball in patients with AMD in hopes that the cells will induce regrowth of the photoreceptors destroyed by the disease.

A similar trial at the Stem Cell Ophthalmology Treatment Study (SCOTS) in Florida is using bone marrow-derived stem cells. In addition Cell Cure Neurosciences has just filed an Investigational New Drug Application with the FDA for a phase I/IIa trial to test the safety and efficacy of their proprietary retinal pigment epithelial cells treatment for AMD. There are no results yet from any of these studies, but 2015 promises to be a very interesting year for AMD.

Retinitis Pigmentosa

ReNeuron, a British company, is using its proprietary human retinal progenitor cells as the basis of its ReN003 therapy targeting retinitis pigmentosa, a group of hereditary diseases of the eye that lead to progressive loss of sight due to cells in the retina becoming damaged and eventually dying.

Three other phase I/II studies are also ongoing: one in India, one in Thailand and one in the United States. All three are using bone marrow derived stem cells.

Glaucoma

We're nowhere near a regenerative cure for glaucoma yet, but some preliminary work has been done. Glaucoma is a leading cause of blindness and is caused by increased pressure inside the eyeball causing the death of fragile retinal ganglion cells (RGCs). Neurotrophic factors (NTFs), which travel along the axon of a neuron to a RGC act as survival signals, but after injury or disease, this supply is lost and RGCs die. Supplementation of injured RGCs with an alternative source of NTFs could protect them from death. Researchers at the University of Birmingham (UK) have found that injecting certain stem cells into the eyes of rats causes the sustained release of NTFs (and other factors) in proximity to damaged RGCs resulting in their survival in the face of traumatic injury.[78]

The implication is that there is a certain cocktail of "factors" that can heal damaged retinal nerve cells before they die and vision becomes permanently impaired. Specialized stem cells may turn out to be the best delivery vehicle for these factors, to ensure that a continuous supply of factors can be applied to damaged cells for a long enough time for them to recover.

Cancer

Cancer is a unique disease in that every patient's cancer is different. Unlike infectious diseases, where a virus or bacteria can usually be targeted by the same therapeutic agent in all patients, cancers are not only much more diverse, but they change with time.

Cancer cells fool the patient's immune system by "camouflaging" themselves. Since every patient is different the camouflage tends also to be different. In addition as the cancer develops it can change its camouflage.

Much of today's cancer research is focusing on the possible solution of "personalizing" a therapeutic agent to each patient's cancer. Frequently this involves "customizing" the patient's own immune system stem cells to produce cancer-specific immune cells which are then injected back into the patient to attack the tumor. Since the patient's own stem cells are used this approach avoids the graft-vs.-host reaction problem, but at the same time it makes the therapy more costly and time consuming.

Typical of this approach is Northwest Biotherapeutics's DCVax® system, which uses immune system stem cells from the blood and cancer tissue samples to mobilize the entire immune system against the target cancer. The company is now running a phase III trial on glioblastoma multiforme (a very deadly brain cancer) and a phase I/II trial on all types of inoperable solid tumors. It has released one case report from the latter trial that showed substantial tumor necrosis (cell death) and initial tumor regression in a sarcoma patient.

Attacking cancers using the immune system is not necessarily the only viable approach. Researchers at Lund University in Sweden recently have proposed a different and innovative way to treat brain (and possibly other) cancers with stem cells.

Neural (i.e. brain) stem cells are attracted to tumor cells in the brain and migrate to their location. If stem cells are injected into one part of the brain and there is a glioma (a brain cancer) in another part of the brain, the stem cells will move to the tumor area. Interestingly, the stem cells seem also to have an innate ability to fight off the tumor cells.

We don't know yet why this happens, but it seems to be a general mechanism. The researchers at Lund also tested the neural stem cells against colon cancers and they worked in those cases too. Obviously a lot of research remains to be done before this information turns into a cancer-fighting therapy. But the basic knowledge that some stem cells can successfully combat cancer opens up a whole new front in regenerative medicine.

Part IV:
The Future of
Regenerative
Medicine

8

Problems and Challenges

Last year the world's first stem cell "drug" was approved and released in Canada. Prochyma (Osiris Therapeutics, Inc.) is a proprietary preparation of bone marrow MSCs (mesenchymal stem cells) which has powerful anti-inflammatory properties. It has passed phase III trials in treatment of graft-vs.-host disease, a complication of bone marrow transplant in children, and is available for approved uses as a prescription drug in Canada. The FDA has approved it for studies in the United States and it is undergoing trials for use in Crohn's disease, COPD, type 1 diabetes, heart attacks and acute radiation syndrome.

This is just the beginning of what we expect to be a cornucopia of stem cell therapies coming over the next years. We have seen above that numerous therapies are on the launching pad. But what are the challenges that new therapies must overcome? We explore the possibilities in the paragraphs below.

Delivery

Currently stem cells must usually be delivered to their destination either surgically or by direct injection into the target tissue. It would save a good deal of time and complicated procedures if a different and better way could be found.

We know that stem cells are attracted to areas of acute inflammation. This is probably how the basic version of prolotherapy works. Since prolotherapy treatments are used for problems easily accessible by needles this approach works well for stem cell prolotherapy with as well.

But how about *in situ* regeneration of internal tissues not easily approachable by needles —heart, liver, pancreas, and others? Right now, the experimental therapies using the *in situ* regeneration approach use a long catheter threaded through major veins to get close enough to the target tissue so that stem cells can be injected directly. These are major procedures requiring a radiology suite and interventional radiologists—time consuming and expensive.

What is needed is an easier way to deliver the stem cells to their target. We are just starting to see intravenously injectable or oral agents developed that target specific tissues or organs. These could be used to attract stem cells to a destination either by attaching the agent to stem cells or by attaching it to a stem-cell attractant. Either way stem cells injected intravenously would then home in on the particular target.

Even further down the line we hope to learn what exactly it is about acute inflammation that attracts and activates stem cells. Once these factors are known the next step will be to figure out how to induce the expression of these factors in target tissues selectively. It may then be possible to attract stem cells to their desired destination and put them to work without resorting to a full-fledged inflammatory reaction.

It seems unlikely that we will ever find a stem cell delivery method that does not involve injection or implantation of some kind. Stem cells are fairly fragile and unlikely to ever be able to get through the GI tract and into the blood, even if encapsulated in some kind of protective barrier. So oral therapies are not very likely in the foreseeable future.

Therapy

Stem cells may be natural, but that doesn't mean that they aren't susceptible to improvement. Current research seems to indicate that sometimes it is not so much the stem cells themselves that are important in the effects on organs and tissues, but the growth factors and chemical signals that stem cells (and platelets) release when activated. It is these factors that cause other stem cells to replicate, forming new tissue, including blood vessels and other supporting structures. Several studies have had successful clinical outcomes and yet found no remaining outside stem cells at the end of the study period. Thus stem cells and platelets may sometimes be mostly just delivery vehicles, rather than actual building blocks of change.

If further research proves that to be the case then we can expect pharmaceutical companies to try to reproduce stem cell effects by using new growth factors. Since growth factors themselves can't be patented (because they are natural substances) the new products probably will be either variations on natural growth-factor molecules (similar to the artificial hormones now produced by drug companies) or bioidentical growth factors manufactured by patented processes. In fact one such growth factor, PDGF (platelet derived growth factor), is already on the market.

But it seems unlikely that growth factors by themselves will be the answer. The processes and milieu in which tissue regeneration takes place is very complex and involves multiple factors, both from the stem cells and from the local environment. It seems more likely that regeneration requires a precise mix of many different growth factors, enzymes, and chemical signals, and quite possibly this mix changes over the time course of healing. Some experiments using cytokines (small signaling molecules that cells use to communicate with their neighbor and internally) from young stem cells in a culture of old stem cells have shown that the young cytokines can cause the old cells to revert to younger gene expression patterns.[79] We might infer from this that optimal regeneration requires a specific sequence of growth factors, cytokines, and other substances delivered in a specific place at a specific time and rate.

So it's likely that we may need the cells after all, if only to act as mixing and dispensing vehicles. But the harvesting and preparation of stem cells is the most time-consuming part of regenerative medicine procedures. It would be really welcomed if we could shorten that step.

Three potential ways to make the stem cell preparation more efficient are artificial stem cells, encapsulated stem cells and antigen-stripped stem cells. One of the main problems of adult stem cells is their immunogenicity. That's why we prefer to use autologous (the patient's own) stem cells—so recipients' immune systems won't reject them or trigger an allergic reaction. Since stem cells are (for our purposes) just vesicles (very, very tiny balloons with a membrane of fat rather than rubber) in which growth factors, cytokines, and perhaps other agents are stored and then released, it should be possible to manufacture such vesicles with non-antigenic membranes. Even better, such artificial stem cells could have custom mixes of growth factors, cytokines, etc., perhaps tailored to purpose.

The antigen-stripping method involves either growing antigen-free stem cells (antigens are the molecules in cell membranes that cause immune reactions) or inducing them and then applying agents or processes to strip the antigens out of the membranes. Such "generic" stem cells could then be banked for immediate use in any patient who needed them.

This is the route being followed by many stem cell companies today. Many of the early successes indicate that such cells are not only possible, but very useful. Bioheart Inc, for instance, has engineered muscle stem cells that have been injected into patients with congestive heart failure, demonstrating excellent results.[80]

At least two research groups are following the encapsulation strategy. In diabetes it's important to have functioning beta cells to produce insulin. Rather than use the patient's own beta cells, which might be difficult to get, these groups have developed ways to implant inert pouches or reservoirs beneath the skin and then fill them with beta cells from their labs. The pouches are made of permeable membranes that allow the insulin produced by the beta cells to diffuse out into the blood and nutrients from the blood to enter and keep the cells alive. However, the membrane prevents the patient's immune system cells from attacking the beta cells inside, so they can continue to produce insulin for a long time. This is pretty close to having a new pancreas, at least for the purposes of insulin and blood sugar regulation.

Genetic Engineering and Stem Cells

A few papers have been published showing that we can even improve upon stem cells' natural properties. Stem cells, like other cells, contain DNA, which controls which proteins the cell produces. Genetic engineering has progressed to the point where we can now insert, remove, and control the expression of individual genes, which, in turn allows control of protein production. This makes possible gene manipulation that can cause overexpression or underexpression of particular proteins.

Sometimes this turns out to be ridiculously easy. A short while ago a group from Edinburgh took very old mice, in which the thymus gland (another part of the immune system) had decreased markedly in function (as usually happens in aging) and changed their DNA to overexpress a single protein that decreases with aging and thus causes a decrease in thymus size and function. Over a period of just a month the increase in this protein caused the thymus stem cells to multiply and the gland to more than double in size and regain much of its youthful capacity.[81]

Bioheart also has combined regenerative medicine with genetic engineering in its second-generation heart stem cells (fig. 31). They have modified the stem cells to overexpress a protein that regulates cell proliferation. When these modified stem cells are injected into failing hearts they seem to grow twice as much new muscle as the first-generation cells did.

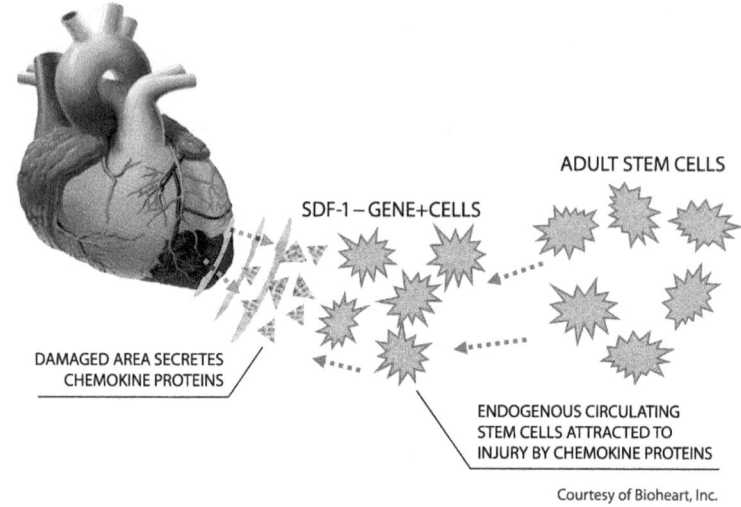

ADULT STEM CELLS

SDF-1 – GENE+CELLS

DAMAGED AREA SECRETES
CHEMOKINE PROTEINS

ENDOGENOUS CIRCULATING
STEM CELLS ATTRACTED TO
INJURY BY CHEMOKINE PROTEINS

Courtesy of Bioheart, Inc.

Figure 31. Heart stem cells improved by gene therapy can produce more heart muscle and a better blood supply.

Another example is sickle cell disease. This common ailment is genetic and causes the victims to produce red blood cells (RBCs) that become deformed, blocking blood flow and causing pain and organ damage. On average, patients survive only into their 40s.

Some people have been cured by bone marrow transplants of genetically normal red blood cells. But of course these transplants must come from other people and therefore all the usual risks and problems of graft rejection and immune reactions apply.

Bad genes, however, are susceptible to genetic engineering. A phase I study is starting now at University of California at Los Angeles in which sickle cell patients will be given marrow transplants of their own bone marrow (thus avoiding graft rejection and immune reactions) —but modified. After the bone marrow sample is taken and before it is reinjected into the patient the researchers will insert a new gene into the DNA of the red blood stem cells, a gene that will prevent the RBCs from sickling. When these cells regenerate the patient's blood supply they will produce normal healthy RBCs and the disease will be cured. It's essentially an autologous organ transplant, in which the blood is the organ.

These examples are very simple, however. The combination of stem cell therapy and genetic engineering is going to get a lot more complicated and powerful. Here is a final example:

OncoCyte, a subsidiary of BioTime, is starting studies to use induced pluripotent potentiated endothelial stem cells to fight cancer. You'll recall that induced pluripotent stem cells (iPSCs) are stem cells that have been made by taking normal cells and "regressing" them backwards into becoming stem cells. Endothelial cells are the cells that line your blood vessels and endothelial stem cells are naturally attracted to areas of developing new blood vessels – such as cancerous tumors.

But these will be specialized endothelial iPSCs. They are genetically engineered iPSCs with new genes inserted which produce specific enzymes. These enzymes convert a harmless prodrug (a molecular precursor to a drug) into a lethal cancer-killing drug. The iPSCs also have a second set of new genes: ones that are programmed to make the cells self-destruct when they get a certain chemical signal.

So the scenario unfolds like this: The genetically engineered endothelial iPSCs are injected into the patient. They home in on the new blood vessels being formed in the cancer tumors and attach themselves there. The prodrug is administered next, and when it encounters an iPSC, the enzymes produced by the new genes inserted into the iPSC DNA convert it into the anti-cancer drug, which kills the surrounding cancer cells. Then the chemical signal drug is given to the patient. It causes all the iPSCs to self-destruct and they are cleared from the body. Two big advantages to this method are that the iPSCs and the prodrug will reach everywhere in the body, so if there is metastatic tumor, it will be treated, regardless of location, and at the end of the treatment all the stem cells will be gone so there is no chance of adverse effects from them.

Regenerative medicine will revolutionize healthcare. Many toxic drug therapies and risky surgical procedures will be replaced by more natural regenerative healing processes. We anticipate that many diseases for which there has been no hope will be routinely cured. In the evolving development of regenerative medicine fortunes may be made and lost and Nobel prizes will be won. In any case we are all fortunate to be living through this revolution.

Appendix: Finding a Practitioner

Since regenerative medicine is such a new specialty there are no formal university training programs yet. Doctors who want to learn regenerative medicine have to get their training piecemeal by going to educational programs for specific techniques. Some residency and fellowship programs include training in some aspects of regenerative medicine. For example, several osteopathic medical programs include prolotherapy in their curricula as does the family medicine residency of the University of Wisconsin.

A number of doctors learn regenerative techniques by the time-honored "apprenticeship" method. They first study the literature and learn all they can. Then they find a doctor who is already skilled in the technique and go observe and assist this mentor in their practice for a while, learning the techniques under their direct supervision.

The closest thing to a comprehensive training program is the fellowship in anti-aging and regenerative medicine offered by the American Academy of Anti-Aging

Medicine (A4M). Even this fellowship falls a little short, however, in that it does not include prolotherapy training.

The American Board of Anti-Aging and Regenerative Medicine (ABAARM) offers a certification examination (that includes both oral and written parts) to physicians who want to test their knowledge and skills in anti-aging and regenerative medicine. This board, however, like a number of other small specialized medical boards, is not a member of the American Board of Medical Specialties. That is, it is not recognized by the mainstream medical establishment.

Below we list the websites of organizations that have lists of members or graduates of their programs in various aspects of regenerative medicine. You can find direct links to the organizations with which our practice is associated on our website: www.rejuvacare.org.

Bioidentical Hormone Replacement Therapy

American Academy of Anti-Aging Medicine (A4M)

http://www.a4m.com/directory.html

Age Management Medical Group (AMMG)

https://www.agemed.org/ActiveAMMEFPhysicianDire ctory/tabid/1163/language/en-US/Default.aspx

Worldlink Medical

http://worldlinkmedical.com/directory/

Forever Health - Suzanne Somers' website for BHRT

https://network.foreverhealth.com/?returnUrl=Doctor Search%2FSearch

Prolotherapy

Hackett-Hemwall Foundation (University of Wisconsin)

http://www.hacketthemwall.org/List_of_Prolotherapist s.html

American Association of Orthopaedic Medicine (AAOM)

http://www.aaomed.org/orthopaedic-doctor

American Osteopathic Association of Prolotherapy Regenerative Medicine (AOAPRM)

http://prolotherapycollege.org/Physicians.php

GetProlo—This website includes a wealth of information about prolotherapy in addition to a list of prolotherapists

http://www.getprolo.com

Stem Cell Therapy

US Stem Cell Training, Inc. (www.usstemcelltraining.com)

Doesn't post a list, but if you send them an email to treatment@bioheartinc.com they will send you the names and contact information for physicians in your area who have been trained in their stem cell techniques.

Ageless Regenerative Institute
http://www.agelesshealth.com/

Also has no list, but will direct you to someone in their network if you ask.

Academy of Regenerative Practices
http://www.regenerativeacademy.com

Has a physician finder program.

A4M (see above) - Doesn't list stem cell training separately, but does list members and physicians who have passed the ABAARM certification examination.

Glossary

adult stem cell - a stem cell which has developed to the point where it is limited in the types of tissue that it can produce.

allogeneic - A transplant where the donated material comes from a different individual than the recipient.

antigen - a substance that binds to an antibody and causes an immune reaction.

antigenic - acting like an antigen.

arthrodesis - the surgical fixation of a joint.

arthroplasty - surgery to realign or reconstruct a joint.

astrocyte - a supporting cell in the brain and spinal cord.

autologous - coming from the same body. Autologous fat is fat taken from one site on a person and then placed into another site on the same person.

cadaveric - from a cadaver or dead body.

cannula - a thin, narrow tube. Like a hypodermic needle except with a blunt tip.

carotid artery - a large blood vessel that supplies the brain.

Cell Medicine, Cellular Medicine - see Regenerative Medicine

chemotherapy - treatment of cancer with anticancer drugs.

cloning - the process of producing similar populations of genetically identical individuals.

collagen - a fibrous protein material that stretches throughout the skin and subcutaneous tissue

cortisone - an anti-inflammatory hormone

cytokines - specialized small molecules that carry a signal within a cell or between cells

delivery system - a method to place a chemical or cell into a desired location

dermis - the second layer of skin, just beneath the epidermis.

differentiate, differentiation - the process by which a stem cell turns into a final tissue cell.

dihydrotestosterone, DHT - a hormone metabolite of testosterone. It suppresses hair growth.

dopamine - a neurotransmitter chemical.

dose escalation trial - a study in which gradually increasing doses of a therapeutic agent are given to determine the threshold and maximum doses.

embryonic stem cell - stem cell that comes from an embryo. The first and most basic of stem cells.

emphysema, chronic obstructive pulmonary disease, COPD - a lung disease defined by persistently poor airflow as a result of breakdown of lung tissue and dysfunction of the small airways.

endothelial - relating to the endothelium, the thin layer of cells that lines the interior surface of blood vessels.

extracellular matrix - the framework that surrounds and supports the cells. Mostly made up of collagen and hyaluronic acid.

facet joints - the joints between spinal vertebra

fibroblast - a connective tissue cell. Fibroblasts produce collagen.

gene therapy - the use of genetic engineering techniques to repair or replace DNA.

genome - the complete set of hereditary factors contained in a set of chromosomes.

granule - a small spherical bag packed with various chemicals that sits within a cell or platelet until called upon. At that point it merges with the cell membrane and empties its chemicals into the extracellular space.

growth factor - A substance that affects the growth of an organism.

growth hormone - A hormone secreted by the pituitary gland that promotes growth of the body.

hemoglobin A1c - hemoglobin A with a glucose molecule attached. It is a measure of the average level of glucose in the blood.

homeostasis - a tendency to equilibrium or stability in the normal physiological states of an organism.

hormone - a natural chemical substance produced in the body which has a specific regulatory effect on the activity of certain cells or a certain organ or organs

hyaluronic acid, HA - a molecule found throughout the skin that absorbs water and thus provides hydration, softness and smoothness.

immunogenicity - the property enabling a substance to provoke an immune response.

immunomodulatory - Capable of modifying or regulating one or more immune functions.

immunosuppress - inhibit or prevent activity of the immune system.

induced pluripotent stem cells (iPSCs) - tissue cells which have been artificially de-differentiated to turn them back into stem cells.

inflammation - the first stage of healng, when stem cells and white blood cells migrate to an injured area.

intra-arterial - inside an artery.

intra-articular - inside a joint.

intradermal - within the skin, usually the dermis

intrathecal - into the spinal canal,

intravenous - inside a vein.

ischemia - a state of insufficient supply of blood to an organ or tissue.

liposuction - the procedure in which subcutaneous fat is sucked out of the body through a small incision.

ligaments - the tough, fibrous bands that run from one bone to another, stabilizing joints and holding the bones in their correct relationship to each other.

megakaryocytic - the cells from which platelets are derived.

mesenchymal stem cells, MSCs - multipotent adult stem cells that can differentiate into a variety of tissues, including bone, muscle, cartilage, fat, etc.

microtubules - long, thin little tubes inside the platelet which act kind of like a skeleton and muscles to maintain and change its shape

monocyte - a type of white blood cell, and therefore part of the immune system.

necrosis - a form of cell injury that results in the premature death of cells.

neurodegenerative - involving degeneration of nerve cells.

neuron - an electrically excitable cell that processes and transmits information through electrical and chemical signals.

neurotransmitter - a chemical used to send a signal from nerve endings.

neurotrophic - inducing the survival, development, and function of neurons.

non-nucleated - without a nucleus, and therefore without most genes

organelle - a specialized subunit within a cell that has a specific function, and it is usually separately enclosed within its own lipid bilayer.

osteoarthritis, OA, DJD, degenerative joint disease - a progressive disorder of the joints caused by gradual loss of cartilage.

osteoporosis - when bones lose an excessive amount of their protein and mineral content, particularly calcium.

pericyte - an adult stem cell that lives on blood vessels

peripheral neuropathy - a wide range of disorders in which the nerves outside of the brain and spinal cord ((peripheral nerves) have been damaged.

peripheral vascular disease, PVD, peripheral arterial occlusive disease, PAOD - the obstruction of large arteries not within the coronary, aortic arch vasculature, or brain.

phase I clinical trial - a study to test the toxicity and/or side effects of a therapy.

phase II clinical trial - a study to determine the appropriate dosage of a therapy

phase III clinical trial - a study to determine the efficacy of a therapy.

physiology - the organic processes or functions in an organism or in any of its parts.

platelets - minute, irregularly shaped, disklike bodies found in blood plasma that promote blood clotting and have no nucleus, no chromosomes, and no hemoglobin.

platelet rich plasma (PRP) - plasma (the liquid part of blood) plus platelets in a greater concentration than normal.

prolotherapy - a method for treating musculoskeletal pain that involves injecting an irritant substance (as dextrose) into a ligament or tendon to promote the growth of new tissue.

radiotherapy - treatment of disease by means of ionizing radiation (x-rays).

regenerative medicine - the process of replacing or regenerating human cells, tissues, or organs to restore or establish normal function.

regression - in a tumor, a decrease in size and/or number of metastases; in a stem cell, a change back to a previous version in the stem cell lineage.

retinal ganglion cells - cells that are part of a retinal ganglion, a nervous structure provide relay points and intermediary connections between different neurological structures.

scaffold - a biologic framework, usually made mainly of collagen, on which stem cells are placed to enhance their ability to form a particular structure.

SCI, spinal cord injury - a traumatic injury to the spinal cord usually resulting in paralysis.

sclerosant - a chemical which causes a scar to form at the site where it is injected.

stem cells - the parent cells from which all other tissue and organ cells are derived.

subcutaneous - underneath the top two layers of skin (dermis and epidermis).

tendons - the tough fibrous bands that attach muscles to bones.

TENS - transcutaneous electrical nerve stimulation. A method for treating pain.

testosterone - the primary male sex hormone (but also present and necessary in women).

therapeutic milieu - the total body environment or conditions in which a therapy takes place.

thyroid hormone - the major hormone regulating the body's metabolism.

transgenic - having genetic material from more than one species.

trophic - the second stage of healing, also called proliferative, when cells divide and organize themselves into new tissue.

tumescent liposuction - a liposuction technique where the subcutaneous tissue is infiltrated with saline and local anesthetic before suctioning.

vesicle - a collection of liquid enclosed by a membrane.

Index

References

[1] Rudman D, Feller AG, Nagrai HS, et al. Effects of human growth hormone in men over 60 years old. *New England Journal of Medicine,* 323(1):1–6, 1990.

[2] Mason C & Dunnil P. A brief definition of regenerative medicine. *Regenerative Medicine,* 3(1):1–5, 2008.

[3] Wartian SP. *HRT, The Answers: A Concise Guide for Solving the Hormone Replacement Therapy Puzzle.* Healthy Living Books, Incorporated, 2003.

[4] Somers S. *Ageless: The Naked Truth about Bioidentical Hormones.* New York, NY: Random House, Inc., 2006.

[5] Wright JV, Lenard L, & Somers S. *Stay Young & Sexy with Bioidentical Hormone Replacement: The Science Explained.* Smart Publications, 2009.

[6] Rouzier N. *How to Achieve Healthy Aging,* 2nd Edition. Worldlink Medical Publishing, 2007.

[7] de Grey A & Rae M. *Ending Aging: The Rejuvenation Breakthroughs that Could Reverse Human Aging in Our Lifetime.* New York, NY: St. Martin's Griffin, 2007.

[8] Miller-Keane & O'Toole M. Megakaryocytes. *Miller-Keane Encyclopedia & Dictionary of Medicine, Nursing & Allied Health,* Revised reprint, 7th edition. Philadelphia, PA: Elsevier, 2005.

[9] Nasiek DJ. *PRP Platelet Rich Plasma: A New Paradigm of Regenerative Medicine.* Island Park, NY: Master Printing USA, 2013. A great book that goes into more detail about how all this happens and how PRP works.

[10] Hackett GS & Henderson DG. Joint stabilization; an experimental, histologic study with comments on the clinical application in ligament proliferation. *Am. J. Surg.*, 89(5):968–73, 1955 May.

[11] Liu YK, Tipton CM, Matthes RD, Bedford TG, Maynard JA, & Walmer HC. An in situ study of the influence of a sclerosing solution in rabbit medial collateral ligaments and its junction strength. Connect Tissue Res. 1983;11(2–3):95–102.

[12] Rabago D, Slattengren A, & Zgierska A. Prolotherapy in primary care practice. Prim Care. 37(1):65–80, doi: 10.1016/j.pop.2009.09.013, 2010 Mar.

[13] Distel LM & Best TM. Prolotherapy: a clinical review of its role in treating chronic musculoskeletal pain. PM R. 3(6 Suppl 1):S78–81, doi: 10.1016/j.pmrj.2011.04.003, 2011 Jun.

[14] Hauser RA & Hauser MA. *Prolo your pain away: Curing chronic pain with prolotherapy,* 2nd ed. Oak Park, IL: Beulah Land Press. 2004.

[15] Darrow, Marc. *Prolotherapy: The Hollywood Pain Solution.* Protex Press, 2003.

[16] George SH. *Ligament and Tendon Relaxation (Skeletal Disability) Treated by Prolotherapy (Fibro-osseous Proliferation).* Charles C. Thomas Publisher, 1958.

[17] *Orthopedics 2.0,* by Christopher J. Centeno, 2013, Regenexx

[18] Sclafani A & McCormick S. Induction of dermal collagenesis, angiogenesis, and adipogenesis in human skin by injection of platelet-rich fibrin matrix. Archives of Facial Plastic Surgery 2013; 14(2):132–26.

[19] Jaslow R. Vampire facials: a spooky sounding way to rejuvenate skin. 2013, Nov 5. [Video file and article]. Retrieved from http://www.cbsnews.com/news/vampire-facials-a-spookysounding-way-to-rejuvenate-skin/

[20] Powell H. *Tried and Tested: The Vampire Facial.* 2011, Jan 1. [Video file and article]. Retrieved from http://www.thenational.ae/lifestyle/wellbeing /tried-and-tested-the-vampire-facial

[21] Runels, Charles. *Vampire Facelift: The Secret Blood Method to Revive Youth & Restore Beauty.* 2013.

[22] Brietzke SE & Mair EA. Injection snoreplasty: How to treat snoring without all the pain and expense. *Otolaryngol Head Neck Surg.* 124(5):503–10, 2001 May.

[23] Dr. John Sessions, personal communication.

[24] Al-Jassim AH & Lesser THJ. Single dose injection snoreplasty: investigation or treatment.. *The Journal of Laryngology & Otology.* 122(11):1190–3, 2008 Nov.

[25] Somers S. *Knockout: Interviews with Doctors Who Are Curing Cancer and How to Prevent Getting It in The First Place.* Chicago: Harmony. 2009.

[26] Sclafani AP & McCormick SA. Induction of dermal collagenesis, angiogenesis, and adipogenesis in human skin by injection of platelet-rich fibrin matrix. *Arch. Facial Plast. Surg.* 2011 Oct 17.

[27] Okabe K et al. Injectable soft-tissue augmentation by tissue engineering and regenerative medicine with human mesenchymal stromal cells, platelet-rich plasma and hyaluronic acid scaffolds. *Cytotherapy,* 11(3):307–16, 2009.

[28] Dr. Charles Runels, personal communication.

[29] Global Stem Cells, Inc., Bioheart, Inc., and Paul Perito Urology Announce Plans to Launch Stem Cell Clinical Trials for Treatment of Erectile Dysfunction (ED), Miami, FL (PRWEB) February 11, 2014.

[30] Dr. Mark Pinell, personal communication.

[31] Gnedeva K, Vorotelyak E, Cimadamore F, Cattarossi G, Giusto E, Terskikh V, Derivation of Hair-Inducing Cell from Human Pluripotent Stem Cells, *PLOS One* January 21, 2015. DOI: 10.1371/journal.pone.0116892.

[32] Hauser RA & Hauser MA. Op.cit.. P. 81 .

[33] Ongley M, Klein R, Dorman T, Eck B & Hubert L. A new approach to the treatment of chronic low back pain. *Lancet*, 2:143–6. 1987.

[34] Liu YK, op. cit.

[35] Dagenais S, Yelland MJ, Del Mar C, & Schoene ML. Prolotherapy injections for chronic low-back pain. *Cochrane Database Syst. Rev.*, 2:CD004059. 2007 Apr 18.

[36] Hauser RA & Hauser MA. Dextrose Prolotherapy for Unresolved Low Back Pain. *A Retrospective Case Series Study Journal of Prolotherapy*, 3:145–55. 2009.

[37] Watson JD & Shay BL. Treatment of chronic low-back pain: A 1-year or greater follow-up. *J. Altern. Complement Med.*, 16(9): 951–8. doi: 10.1089/acm.2009.0719. 2010 Sep.

[38] Beckworth J. Safety and Preliminary Efficacy Study of Mesenchymal Precursor Cells (MPCs) in Subjects With Lumbar Back Pain, NCT01290367., Emory Orthopaedics & Spine Center.

[39] Reeves KD & Hassanein K. Randomized, prospective, placebo-controlled double-blind study of dextrose prolotherapy for osteoarthritic thumb and finger (DIP, PIP, and trapeziometacarpal) joints: evidence of clinical efficacy. *J. Altern. Complement Med.*, 6(4):311–20. 2000 Aug.

[40] Hauser RA, Ostergaard S, & Santilli S. Stabilization of Rheumatoid Thumb Interphalangeal Joint Boutonniere Deformity and Severe Subluxation with Splinting and Prolotherapy. A Case Report. *Journal of Prolotherapy*, 4:e849–54. 2012.

[41] Rotator Cuff Shoulder Injuries, *The Townsend Letter*. 361–2:114. 2013. Aug/Sep.

[42] Ben-Galim P, Steinberg EL, Amir H, Ash N, Dekel S, & Arbel R. Accuracy of magnetic resonance imaging of the knee and unjustified surgery. *Clin. Orthop. Relat. Res.* 447:100–4. 2006 Jun.

[43] Centeno CJ, Busse D, Kisiday J, Keohan C, Freeman M, & Karli D. Increased knee cartilage volume in degenerative joint disease using percutaneously implanted, autologous mesenchymal stem cells. *Pain Physician*, 11(3):343–53, ISSN: 1533-3159. 2008 May–Jun.

[44] Li H, Seon JK, Hacker M, Franz S, & Simon JC. Mesenchymal Stem Cells in Cartilage Regeneration. *Current Stem Cell Research & Therapy*, ISSN: 1574-888X. 2014 Jul 9.

[45] David R, Jeffrey JP, Marlon M, Richard KJG, Neil AS, Aleksandra Z. Dextrose Prolotherapy for Knee Osteoarthritis: A Randomized Controlled Trial. *Ann. Fam. Med.*, 11:229–237. 2013. doi: 10.1370/afm.1504.

[46] Rabago D, Patterson JJ, Mundt M, Zgierska A, Fortney L, Grettie J, & Kijowski R. Dextrose and morrhuate sodium injections (prolotherapy) for knee osteoarthritis: a prospective open-label trial. *J. Altern. Complement Med.*, 20(5):383–91. 2014 May. doi: 10.1089/acm.2013.0225. Epub 2014 Mar 17.

[47] Patel S, Dhillon MS, Aggarwal S, Marwaha N, & Jain A. Treatment With Platelet-Rich Plasma Is More Effective Than Placebo for Knee Osteoarthritis: A Prospective, Double-Blind, Randomized Trial. *Am. J. Sports Med.* 2013 Jan 8.

[48] Halpern B, Chaudhury S, Rodeo SA, Hayter C, Bogner E, Potter HG, & Nguyen J. Clinical and MRI Outcomes After Platelet – Rich Plasma Treatment for Knee Osteoarthritis. *Clinical Journal of Sport Medicine*, 23(3):238–9. 2013 May.

[49] Mishra A & Pavelko T. Treatment of chronic elbow tendinosis with buffered platelet-rich plasma. *Am. J. Sports Med.*, 34(11):1774–8. Epub 2006 May 30. 2006 Nov.

[50] Michalek J et al, Autologous Adipose Tissue-Derived Stromal Vascular Fraction Cells Application In Patients With Osteoarthritis, *Cell Transplantation* CT-1300 accepted 9 Jan 15 for publication doi: 10.3727/096368915X686760

[51] Hernigou P et al. Osteonecrosis repair with bone marrow cell therapies: State of the clinical art. *Bone.* 2015 Jan; 70:102-9. doi: 10.1016/j.bone.2014.04.034. Epub 2014 Jul 10.

[52] Brian Shiple, DO, personal communication.

[53] Say F, Türkeli E, & Bülbül M. Is platelet-rich plasma injection an effective choice in cases of non-union? *Acta Chir Orthop Traumatol Cech.* 2014;81(5):340-5.

[54] Bielecki T, Gazdzik TS, & Szczepanski T. Benefit of percutaneous injection of autologous platelet-leukocyte-rich gel in patients with delayed union and nonunion. *Eur Surg Res.* 2008;40(3):289-96. doi: 10.1159/000114967. Epub 2008 Feb 15.

[55] Qu Z, Mi S, & Fang G., Clinical study on treatment of bone nonunion with MSCs derived from human umbilical cord, *Zhongguo Xiu Fu Chong Jian Wai Ke Za Zhi.* 2009 Mar;23(3):345-7.

[56] Reurink G, Goudswaard GJ, et al. Platelet-Rich Plasma Injections in Acute Muscle Injury. *N. Engl. J. Med.,* 370:2546–47, 2014 DOI: 10.1056/NEJMc1402340. 2014 June 26.

[57] Hsieh MM, Fitzhugh CD, Weitzel RP, Link ME, Coles WA, Zhao X, Rodgers GP, Powell JD, & Tisdale JF. Nonmyeloablative HLA-matched sibling allogeneic hematopoietic stem cell transplantation for severe sickle cell phenotype. *JAMA: The Journal of The American Medical Association [JAMA],* ISSN: 1538-3598, 312(1):48–56. 2014 Jul 2.

[58] Schloendorf J. *Life Extension Magazine.,* p44. January 2014.

[59] Procházka V et al. Cell Therapy, a New Standard in Management of Chronic Critical Limb Ischemia and Foot Ulcer. *Cell Transplantation*, 19(11):1413–24. 2010 7 June.

[60] Jonsson TB, Larzon T, Arfvidsson B, Tidefelt U, Axelsson CG, Jurstrand M, & Norgren L. Adverse events during treatment of critical limb ischemia with autologous peripheral blood mononuclear cell implant. *Int Angiol*, (1):77–84. 2012 Feb 31.

[61] Linyi P, Zhuqing J, et al. Comparative Analysis of Mesenchymal Stem Cells from Bone Marrow, Cartilage, and Adipose Tissue. *Stem Cells and Development*, 17(4):761–74. 2008 Aug. doi: 10.1089/scd.2007.0217.

[62] ClinicalTrials.gov Identifier: NCT02099500.

[63] Comella K, et al., Clinical Applications of Adipose Derived Stem Cells. *ISSCR Poster Session* 2012, Japan.

[64] DashSurjya N, DashNihar R, GuruBhikaricharan, & Mohapatra Prakash C. *Rejuvenation Research* 17(1):40–53. 2014 Feb. doi: 10.1089/rej.2013.1467.

[65] Rinkevich Y et al. In Vivo Clonal Analysis Reveals Lineage-Restricted Progenitor Characteristics in Mammalian Kidney Development, Maintenance, and Regeneration. *Cell Rep*, pii: S2211–1247(14)00305–2. May 14. doi: 10.1016/j.celrep.2014.04.018. 2014.

[66] Personal communication Drs. J Perez and J Lopez, Regenerative Medicine Institute, Tijuana, Mexico.

[67] Tzouvelekis A, Ntolios P, & Bouros D. Stem cell treatment for chronic lung diseases. *Respiration*, 85(3):179–92. 2013. doi: 10.1159/000346525. Epub 2013 Jan 29.

[68] Iman SB, Armand K, & Robert PG. Concise Review: Bone Marrow Autotransplants for Liver Disease?. *Stem Cells*, 31(11):2313–29, 2013 Nov.

[69] Bright R, Bright M, Bright P, Hayne S, & Thomas WD. Migraine and Tension-Type Headache Treated With Stromal Vascular Fraction: A Case Series. *J Med Case Reports*, 8(237). 2014.

[70] Shruster A & Offen D. Targeting neurogenesis ameliorates danger assessment in a mouse model of Alzheimer's disease. *Behav. Brain Res.* 261:193–201. 2014 Mar 15. doi: 10.1016/j.bbr.2013.12.028. Epub 2013 Dec 31.

[71] Proschel C, Stripay JL, Shih CH, Munger JC, & Noble MD. Delayed transplantation of precursor cell-derived astrocytes provides multiple benefits in a rat model of Parkinsons. *EMBO Mol Med*, [Epub ahead of print] 2014 Jan 29.

[72] Thomsen GM, Gowing G, Svendsen S, & Svendsen CN. The past, present and future of stem cell clinical trials for ALS. *Exp. Neurol.* pii: S0014-4886(14)00073-9. 2014 Mar 6. doi: 10.1016/j.expneurol. 2014.02.021. [Epub ahead of print].

[73] Chen L, Coleman R, et al. "Human Neural Precursor Cells Promote Neurologic Recovery in a Viral Model of Multiple Sclerosis. *Stem Cell Reports.* http://dx.doi.org/10.1016/j.stemcr.2014.04.005

[74] Riordan NH, Ichim TE, Min WP, Wang H, Solano F, Lara F, Alfaro M, Rodriguez JP, Harman RJ, Patel AN, Murphy MP, Lee RR, & Minev B. Non-expanded adipose stromal vascular fraction cell therapy for multiple sclerosis. *J Transl Med*, 7:29. 2009.

[75] van Gorp S et al. Amelioration of motor/sensory dysfunction and spasticity in a rat model of acute lumbar spinal cord injury by human neural stem cell transplantation. *Stem Cell Research & Therapy*, 4:57–79. 2013.

[76] Lu P et al. Long-distance growth and connectivity of neural stem cells after severe spinal cord injury. *Cell,* 150(6):1264–73. 2012.

[77] Lv YT, et al. Transplantation of human cord blood mononuclear cells and umbilical cord-derived mesenchymal stem cells in autism. *J Transl Med*, 11:196. 2013 Aug 27.

[78] Mead B, Logan A, Berry M, Leadbeater W, & Scheven BA. Dental pulp stem cells, a paracrine-mediated therapy for the retina. *Neural Regen*, Res, 9:577–8. 2014.

[79] Shane R, Crain A, Golovko A, Morpurgo B, et al. Propitious Modulation of Fibroblast Quiescence Mediated by Cytokine Expression Mediated from Embryonic Stem Cells. *Chapter 16, Anti-Aging Therapeutics*, XV, American Academy of Anti-Aging Medicine. 2014.

[80] Povsic TJ et al. A double-blind, randomized, controlled, multicenter study to assess the safety and cardiovascular effects of skeletal myoblast implantation by catheter delivery in patients with chronic heart failure after myocardial infarction. *Am Heart J.* 2011 Oct;162(4):654-662.e1. doi: 10.1016/j.ahj.2011.07.020. Epub 2011 Sep 9.

[81] Nicholas B, Craig SN, & Clare C. Blackburn Regeneration of The Aged Thymus By A Single Transcription Factor. *Development*, 141:1627–37, 2014 April.

About the Author

Theodore E. Harrison is the author of the books *Computer Billing for Medical/Dental Offices* and *Cruise Medicine* and of numerous articles in the medical literature. He received his B.A. and M.D. degrees from Washington University in St. Louis and did his residency in Emergency Medicine at the Johns Hopkins Hospital in Baltimore.

Dr. Harrison practiced emergency and critical care medicine for several decades before becoming interested in the newly emerging field of anti-aging and regenerative medicine. He retrained and in 2005 became one of a small cadre of physicians to become board-certified in this new (and as of yet unofficial) specialty. He is the co-founder of the Rejuvacare PC Regenerative Medicine Practice in Port Angeles, Washington.

www.ingramcontent.com/pod-product-compliance
Lightning Source LLC
Chambersburg PA
CBHW051914170526
45168CB00001B/390